THE LAZY BEEFEATER'S GUIDE TO HEALTH & WEIGHT LOSS!

WITHOUT GOING HUNGRY

OR GOING TO THE GYM!

BY
DEAN MONCHO

Love
you

CONTENTS

"The Royal Bodyguards of the British monarch were given a very large ration of beef, given to them daily, and so became known as 'Beefeaters'. Beefeaters also commonly produced and consumed broths made of beef, which were described as rich and hearty."

Ask yourself why!

INTRODUCTION

This book is a natural response to a number of friends asking me to talk them through how I lost my gut, got healthy, and did it without going to the gym and without following a restrictive diet. I was eating bacon and eggs and steak for dinner, and more importantly maintaining and keeping the weight off for over two years – to make this my new 'normal'. It's nothing more than an extension of a simple plan of attack, that addresses a problem that has now become the new 'norm' for nearly 75% of the population … the problem of being overweight or obese (and all the health effects that come with it). I am also writing this in the post Covid-19 pandemic where ill health is being punished like never before. If ever you wanted clear proof that an underlying condition increases your susceptibility to an early death, look no further. Pre-existing conditions as defined by the World Health Organisation include obesity, diabetes and smoking.

I would describe myself as objectively average! And not in a bad way. Average in my levels of discipline, average in my levels of activity, and so on. That is to say I'm not at the extreme of, at one end, a 'lost cause' who might need a forklift to get them out of the house; nor at the other extreme of someone who runs marathons and follows a restrictive dietary regime with endless counting and scientific fervour.

I, like most, have had a history of dabbling with different diets and exercise approaches for many years. Not out of some great dissatisfaction with myself, but more from a perspective of slowing a downhill slide of old age culminating in ill health. I've experimented with everything from juicing to Atkins, from the weight room to the hot yoga room. My view is that none of these things in isolation can be a magic bullet – unless taken to an extreme.

So what's missing? The answer is a multi-strategy approach that goes beyond the old simplification of 'diet and exercise'. Like a business, we need to attack an issue from all sides and with multiple strategies. We need to manage the transition to ensure the solution endures, and the results continue to thrive. It is a problem which we all face and which we universally seem to fail at, while following a one-solution strategy. We all seem to hang our hat on a fad diet or a renewed exercise push or regime.

Of course it makes perfect sense that we are more likely to achieve lasting results by combining our efforts and compounding the results from one approach with a kicker from another approach, while attacking an issue on all fronts. The alternative is a bit like treating a common flu with a Paracetamol tablet alone! If we combine sleep, a long bath, vitamin C, Echinacea and good ol' chicken broth etc, we will give our system a much better fighting chance.

Even though I'd been periodically dodging processed white carbs for a while, and going okay, things were hit and miss. Social events, the odd bottle of wine, a bag of sweets … all made for an 'on-again, off-again' approach. Something was missing and I wasn't getting the results I was looking for. However after a motorcycle crash and a neck injury, I fell off the wagon – seemingly for good. Pain medication soon led to alcohol and carbs and earlier progress was mostly lost. Things went downhill fast.

So this book looks to address a few basic practical and psychological issues which, in my view, can get in the way: 1. Simplicity; 2. Ease of nutrition; and 3. Habit-forming routines.

The good news is that by changing not very much at all, you'll turn around your health and your waistline. All this without going hungry, and without going to the gym … starting from ZERO! Assuming you are roughly three stone, 20 kilograms or 50 pounds overweight, have zero fitness, and have tried so-called 'eating healthy' to no avail.

Anyway, let's start with why we want to do this …

Let's start with a wake-up call! You know how we are all worried about climate change and stuff. Yeah well, you have bigger problems! If you're 50 (like me) or over, the way you're going, you'll be lucky to have 10 summers left – so whether the ice-caps melt and mankind is wiped out in a mere 25 years will be irrelevant; because you'll be dead! Covid-19 update: If you are over 60 and have underlying bad health, you're at significantly higher risk of death.

Let's look at some of the statistics if you are an 'average' person living in a developed nation.

Obesity

Obesity is a leading preventable cause of death worldwide, with increasing rates in adults and children. About 40% of middle-aged adults aged 40 to 60 years in developed western nations are obese, and a whopping 75% are considered overweight. Additionally the obesity figures rise to 50% if you are female in that age bracket, which is especially significant with the change in hormones and metabolism which compound almost every aspect. Authorities view obesity as one of the most serious public health problems of the 21st century. Obesity-related conditions include heart disease, stroke, Type2 diabetes and certain types of cancer that are some of the leading causes of preventable and premature death. Conservative predictions are that the problem is only getting worse … much worse! And now this is compounded by Covid-19, with obesity recognised as a contributory risk factor.

High Blood Pressure

Roughly one in every three adults in developed nations have high blood pressure or hypertension. It is slightly more frequent in men and low socioeconomic groups; and it becomes more common with age. Hypertension is the most important preventable risk factor for premature death worldwide. It increases the risk of heart disease, strokes, vascular disease and other cardiovascular diseases including heart attacks, aneurysms, atherosclerosis, kidney disease, atrial fibrillation and pulmonary embolism. Hypertension is also a risk factor for dementia.

Cardiovascular diseases (CVD) or Heart Disease

CVD includes coronary artery diseases (CAD) such as angina and myocardial infarction (commonly known as a heart attacks). Other CVDs include stroke, heart failure, hypertensive heart disease, rheumatic heart disease, cardiomyopathy, abnormal heart rhythms, congenital heart disease, valvular heart disease, aortic aneurysms, peripheral artery disease, thromboembolic disease and venous thrombosis. It is estimated that up to 90% of CVDs may be preventable. Prevention of CVDs involves minimising exposure to risk factors through nutrition, exercise, avoiding smoking and limiting alcohol.

Cardiovascular diseases are the leading cause of death globally. In developed nations, about 40% of us in the age bracket of 40 to 60 years have some form of cardiovascular disease.

Arse cancer

Colorectal cancer, colon cancer, bowel cancer – call it what you will – is the development of cancer from the colon or rectum (parts of the large intestine).

Signs and symptoms may include blood in your poo, changes in bowel movements, weight loss, and feeling tired all the time. Most colorectal cancers are due to old age and lifestyle factors, with only a small number of cases due to underlying genetic disorders. Other risk factors include poor diet, obesity, smoking and lack of physical activity. Dietary factors that increase the risk include processed meats and other processed foods, and alcohol.

Alzheimer's and Dementia

The number of people living with dementia is estimated to double every 20 years. Rates of dementia increase exponentially with increases in age, doubling with every 6.3-year increase in age. A number of factors can decrease the risk of dementia. A group of efforts is believed to be able to prevent one-third of cases and includes early education, treating high blood pressure, preventing obesity, preventing hearing loss, treating depression, being active, preventing diabetes, not smoking, and preventing social isolation. The decreased risk with a healthy lifestyle is seen even in those with a high genetic risk. Also there are fascinating effects of cholesterol, and it's not what you think ... the research shows that people with LOW overall cholesterol are more at risk of brain-degenerative diseases, however we will talk about strategies to increase good cholesterol (HDL) and get the bad stuff like triglycerides and bad cholesterol (LDL) where they should be. Oh boy! The writing's on the wall!

This is NOT a book about some arbitrary external measure such as a six-pack or getting into some dress size. There are easier ways to manage a mid-life crisis. In truth, this book comes from the standpoint that the above conditions and the factors leading to them are more likely to take your life or severely impact it through ill health – more than anything else.

The poor health conditions listed all have something in common: They are all largely preventable through a change in lifestyle – primarily being how and what you eat, and how you exercise. Quite apart from the superficial external appearance of health, this is literally a life-and-death issue if you are in the danger zone of 40 to 60 years old and carrying an extra 30% or more of your optimal body weight.

The top 10 causes of death are:

1. **Heart Disease**
2. **Cancer**
3. **Lung Disease**
4. **Stroke**
5. **Accidents**
6. **Alzheimer's**
7. **Diabetes**
8. **Kidney Disease**
9. **Infections**
10. **Suicide (let's call this one 'poor mental health')**

This book is aimed at tackling these obvious factors standing in your way, which will easily carve 20 years off your lifespan and more than likely greatly impact your quality of life after the age of 50 (and progressively moreso, the older you get).

For your modern-day average Joe or Jane (including my previous self), averagely unhealthy, subject to a good dose of neglect, enduring work stress and a swag of family commitments, time-poor, and with all the other pressures of modern-day life that have taken you from the path of being where you know you should be, you have a recipe for disaster in the long term … at least if you're being honest with yourself. If you don't think you qualify, just take a look at your gut or spare tyre! More than half of us will be far from our youthful prime. We'll have aches and pains and clothes that are tight (or perhaps we've given in and bought looser outfits).

However, as previously mentioned, this book is not aimed at the two extremes of the bell curve. It is not for super-motivated individuals who have a high metabolism, immortal genes and generally more blessings than they are reasonably entitled to; or for those at the other end of the spectrum who have been struck by chronic illness or misfortune which frankly is beyond the remit of a book like this (there is no substitute for the doctor).

For most of us, I believe we have the ability to 'heal thyself'. Indeed those folk who despite their bulging waists, smoking and drinking habits and shortness of breath think that they'll be fine (because 'life is too short') fall into the category of 'health deniers'.

Furthermore, this book is not something that is intended to be dictatorial, or innately critical. We are all human, we all have our vices; so let's not name this 'fat shaming' – but let's call it out and name it 'health shaming'. Ignoring your own wellbeing is not good for you, or your family, or society in general for that matter.

If you're like me, you don't like being told what to do. So take this as a guide, a tip, a hint, a handbook, something to provide a trajectory and a compass heading. Something you can orient yourself by, and navigate back to when needed. Use it to adapt and adopt new habits, and to help you compensate with other strategies if you are struggling in one area or another.

In fact, it's a good general principle in life to stop telling people what to do. So on the premise that everyone is different, if you are pursuing health and wellbeing in your own calm and holistic way and you are perfectly happy with yourself … then great! This book is intended to introduce new ideas, which may complement your own efforts on your path forward. But be honest! If your weekly meditation (or buying organic kale) is providing an excuse for other poor physical health choices, then wake up to the consequences.

This book is a culmination and result of the principles of all the diets, eating plans and exercise plans etc that have worked (and that, equally, haven't worked) 'in isolation' for me. The idea is to take the best bits that work and make sense; and ditch the bits that don't because they are too rigid, unsustainable or too ambitious. We can go through and cherry-pick the best bits that work and ditch the rest. We can then adopt the best features through a key element to making all this work – which is 'gradual transition and adaptation'.

This book also looks at the surrounding factors which keep us from achieving a healthy mind and body – including the excuses and mental constructs that we use as get-out clauses. So what are the four steps and stages that are key to unlocking a permanent solution?

They are:
- **A progressively increasing low carbohydrate way of eating *without* going hungry**

- **A progressively increasing use of Intermittent and therapeutic fasting**

- **A progressive increase of 'gentle' exercise – without pain or injury**

- **A use of slow transitioning to adopt permanent changes, and a non-restrictive mindset**

Once you have made that commitment to change direction (no matter how small) then the benefits will compound – and before you know it, you'll be shopping for smaller clothes in the knowledge that your visceral fat (around your waistline and organs) is leaving the house for good!

Being coachable

Invite yourself to be open-minded and objective. Your greatest experiments and achievements are always fundamentally based on a sample of 'one' and finding what works for you. A really good trait to begin with is the idea that you can be contributed to, and having an open mind. You could call this 'being coachable'.

This book is not meant to be a scientific paper for proof of the benefits of these strategies. There is plenty of reading and empirical proof of the benefits of each of these strategies, and if you want to 'read up' you can go for it (see the further reading section). It's a fascinating and never-ending journey which hopefully begins here. I've put links to further research and sources to elaborate further on the conclusions set out here, but this book is meant to be a practical guide.

Micro-habits

I'm a fan of getting yourself going, finding your mojo, whatever you want to call it … BUT the main mistake (that so many people make) is making grand plans with big targets to achieve huge transformations.

Of course with big plans come big disappointments, and over-ambitious targets seem too far away – so you lose motivation almost as fast as you shared your dreams with those you confided in. The New Year's Resolution syndrome repeats itself all throughout the year! Put simply, we are all lured in by making 'ambitions' rather than making 'changes'. No-one says 'this year I want to be one kilo lighter'; rather everyone wants to squeeze into their wedding dress or have a six-pack like Brad Pitt.

Yet, if we make a small achievable goal, we can quickly set another one – bolstered by a sense of modest achievement. So the key is to make small changes, and let the big ones look after themselves. This coincides with the scientifically documented principle called 'micro-habiting'. Terms like 'creatures of habit' or 'muscle memory' all are testament to the enduring power of habit-forming traits in human beings.

Micro-habiting works on the principle that we are far more likely to maintain a new behaviour when we attach it to an existing behaviour. I won't go into detail about how it's proven, because again there is a heap of science behind this and there is a great TED Talk on the subject – just YouTube the TED Talk on micro-habiting and you'll get it – but in summary it goes like this: Let's say that for the last 10 years you've had 15 chocolate croissants and 10 cups of coffee for breakfast and you can't for the life of you work out why you're fat and anxious with irritable bowel syndrome. Well, once you work it out, you want to change that behaviour … but how? It's a pretty entrenched habit, and you like your breakfast. In fact you'll probably proudly announce that you can't live without your fix. The worst thing you can do is stop cold turkey. It won't last; you'll obsess about your coffee and choccy fix, and BANG you'll be right back to where you started (probably even moreso because, having deprived yourself of what you love, you want it even more). Sound familiar?

The solution is to take your old habit and attach a new habit to it, and make small incremental changes to your existing habit. So this might look like you have nine cups of coffee, but then you have one glass of water and do a 'reminder action' to cement the fact that you have executed the change. This will wean you off an old habit, but fill the void with a reinforced new habit. It might sound like a mind-numbingly obvious statement, that we should replace bad habits with good ones … but in reality the nudge to start with a small habit will break the barrier so we can scratch away at the underlying problem, which is that we are innately resistant to change. Larger habit changes follow smaller ones.

Be as creative as you like, use your imagination and have a bit of fun (in your brain if nowhere else). Once you've had your new amended habit in place for as long as you like, add an element and subtract an element: Subtract the bad stuff like croissants and add good stuff like a push-up … you can do ONE push-up, even if it's off your knees or off the wall? The point is it doesn't matter how small the change is or how long it takes to introduce another change. This is not a race. This is a transformation and there is no time limit; however action is required, no matter how small. Wishing alone won't make things happen.

WHEN YOU PRAY, MOVE YOUR FEET!

AFRICAN PROVERB

Goal setting

Setting goals works for some people as a motivational target, but for other people the mere presence of a fixed goal is a major disincentive as well as a huge set-up for disappointment should they fail to meet a goal within the expected time frame. That is because expectation breeds disappointment. Of course we all accept that we have aspirations, so we tend to dream big and then fail in the same proportion. So what's the answer? Dream small? Well, kind of …

The answer is making small incremental goals. Dream about losing half a kilo! Dream of saving $10! Make a goal of cleaning the sock draw! They are inconsequential, but the process of achieving small targets avoids disappointment and at the same time creates a sense of achievement and completion. What we are doing is starting small and building momentum. However slow, however small, this approach also removes all obstacles to making a start.

In Spain they have a saying 'poco-a-poco' or 'little by little', and in its best interpretation this creates a sense of unpressurised progress. No big goals, just a series of small achievable ones. It's more helpful to set a goal of maintaining a micro-habit such as a 10-minute everyday stretching routine, or 'I won't smoke on Tuesdays', than a distant goal such as 'I want to quit smoking altogether' or 'I want to run a marathon'. People can be so focused on a clearly defined goal that they make no room for transition. In addition we should make room for 'maintenance' as a goal in itself! For example: 'I'm going to lose five kilograms and maintain it for a month'.

There are plenty of successful diet and exercise books out there that attempt a somewhat rigid approach to creating a micro-habit – such as the 80/20 diet, and a few others. They sound good in principle. However, they are lacking in something because they are restrictive and inflexible. They don't give us a path to transition from our existing behaviours to our new ones. In addition they don't allow for when we might stray from the plan, and they give us no way of adapting. It's an 'on-again/off-again' mindset; and we need something better.

These approaches are set up to fail for the vast majority of us, again excluding the 10% who have natural self discipline and therefore don't need a book at all (and the opposite 10% who are genuinely beyond being helped or aren't open to change).

One might eat well during the week and blow out for the weekend; however this type of approach sets up too much variation from a consistent norm to be maintainable. In addition if you're following a low-carb eating plan, which relies heavily on remaining in a state of ketosis, it will take you two or three days to get back into ketosis. An 80/20 rule is a good proportion for life generally for many things – but it doesn't help build consistent changes in behaviour, as consistency is the key.

Instead, if you have a cheat or deviation, it's better to view it as a traffic diversion. Yes, you're off the path, but you make your way back to it and additionally compensate with other strategies. These deviations will always occur and it's no good trying to resist them, or feel guilty or adopt a mindset that you've 'failed'. Otherwise you will not see a small setback as a diversion, but rather an insurmountable obstacle. Work, travel, holidays, special social events, will all throw the odd challenge at you but it's the ability to quickly snap back to your normal habit, or balance through other strategies, that will see true transformation keep hold. It also serves to reduce repetitiveness, as you are not reliant on one thing alone.

With confidence you can traverse these periods and bounce straight back. These are tough as they take you away from your normal (amended or not) routine; and your food choices, routines and opportunities to exercise are thrown into the air. For example, don't bother trying to stay carb-free on a trip to Italy on a gelato/pizza summer break. Nor is it possible to maintain an exercise routine if you're traversing airports, hotels and time-zones and you're exhausted and under pressure. What's the point? Now, if you have a toxic lifestyle where you are constantly travelling, you might have to get a bit more creative. If these are your permanent states of being you have to seriously look at your routines and adapt accordingly. It's not impossible … just harder.

When you take on a 'work-around' approach to your destination, any diversions are soon cancelled out as you get back to your new normal. Three or four kilos from a holiday or business trip are just as quickly shed, because that is what your body naturally wants to do … snap back to normal and get back on track!

So we'll be applying this principle of micro-habits to all the following topics, and alongside detailing a few personal insights in my own journey. I'm 50 years old – I'm now adequately fit, physically and mentally (well I try anyway), and over the last few years I have shed 30 kilograms and kept them off over a period of two years. I've recovered from injury, and recovered my pre-injury weight and fitness; and maintained good health, free from any medication. That is to say, nobody is perfect (especially not me); but no-one should accept hitting middle age with a belly and a packet of biscuits or corn chips – and it's far too easy to allow that to happen through complacency! So let's get on with it.

Here's what we're going to do:

1. A Self-Audit to take stock of where we are right now
2. Work out a plan of attack
3. Address our way of eating
4. Introduce fasting routines
5. Get active and get moving (by the way, No Gym)
6. Put it all together

Disclaimer: A quick word on sources and references and all that. We live in an age of Google, YouTube, TED Talks etc and I am not a scientist – I'm a regular guy with some personal experience and personal research to share. So all of my statements are MY assertions … guesstimates, and probable truths. I probably don't even remember where I heard most things but that doesn't make them less useful. If they resonate with you then that's enough. I will quote some of what I've found useful and where to look to find more. If you feel the need to fact-check or contradictg something with alternate scientific data or contrary views, then go ahead … draw your own conclusions. However you will have missed the point of this book, which is to chill out, take a community view to a different way of eating and staying healthy, and view things with flexibility and move gradually in the right direction towards your goal. Before you know it you will have cemented all three branches of this lifestyle approach, and when they are applied together there's an absolute guarantee of true health, a slim waistline and improved mental clarity and focus.

OKAY, LETS GO!

CHAPTER 1

SELF-AUDIT - LET'S GET REAL!

How do you know where you want to go, if you don't know where you are? Objective self-assessment is essential. This is also important to gain a measure across all areas, including mood, sleep, motivation, libido, etc. It's very easy to assume that we are not making progress because we are not aware of small incremental improvements – but when taken across time, the transformation can be much more noticeable. Plus, you may not feel you are making progress in one area such as a measurement or difference on the scales, whilst dismissing the other areas where you feel great (such as mood or energy levels).

Tale of the tape

It's always hard to believe, but you are about to make some dramatic progress – so it's worth having some baseline measurements to compare yourself to and revisit every three to six months. In essence, do a self-audit! Also, if you are battling any significant medical issues this is the time to visit the doctor and make sure you are not exposing yourself to any undue medical risks for your individual situation.

The things you want to measure are:

- **Weight,** obviously;
- **Blood pressure**;
- **Pulse** – both resting and active [1];
- **Waist circumference** (while you're there why not measure your thigh and upper arm/bicep circumference too);
- **Glucose** – (HbA1c and HS-CRP which are measures to indicate your short-term and average glucose levels and indicate your risk for diabetes/pre-diabetes [2]; and
- **Cholesterol** [3] and Triglycerides.
- **Selfies** – take a couple of selfies (no sucking it in) front-on and profile.

[1] An active pulse reading is to take a reading after about 45 seconds of vigorous exercise such as running on the spot. You then take another reading after the first, keeping very still, and you get a reading which indicates your heart's ability to recover. Resting pulse is also highly sensitive to movement etc, so take it after remaining completely still. A doctor will perform this for you as part of a standard 'physical'.

2 Glucose levels will become irrelevant when you achieve a no-sugar, low to zero carb state; however this is about establishing where you are to start with, and if you are in a pre-diabetic state.

3 Cholesterol comes in many forms but basically you have good cholesterol (HDL) and bad cholesterol (LDL). Increasingly there is a lot of research showing that cholesterol levels are highly influenced by genetics – so it's good to establish what your baseline readings are. Don't panic; overall cholesterol will look high as you adapt to a fat-fuelled diet. Cholesterol can be an alarmist subject, but you should be aware that low levels of cholesterol are linked to increased risk of degenerative brain conditions such as Alzheimer's and stroke. So while cholesterol is important, it needs to be taken in the context of you as an individual. The balance of good versus bad is important, but probably more important are triglycerides.

Generally speaking you want to be lowering bad 'bio indicators', and you should have a think about your physical and mental condition beyond what the bathroom scales look like – regardless of how you stand on them.

Remember that what's on the inside is actually more important than what's on the outside, even if your outward appearance does or doesn't bother you that much. However we are all affected with insecurities and that's normal enough. If you have a spare tyre around your waist, try to visualise the equivalent amount of fat surrounding your organs, surrounding your heart and making it work harder when you run or climb a flight of stairs! Apart from your cardio-vascular system, think about your bad back, your aching knees and all your other aches and pains which go with carrying an extra 30 kilos (five stone or 60 pounds) or more around on your skeletal frame.

Start by noting what your weight was when you were at your ideal weight (by the way, it doesn't matter if you've never been at your ideal weight). Now take the weight difference, and think of that in a suitcase. Yes, the big one that the airline wants you to weigh … yeah, that one! For me personally my excess weight was about 30 kilos when I started this process. We've all struggled to pick up that suitcase and lift it onto the airline scales, yet it seems completely normal that we should carry that around with us every day on our bones, our joints, our backs, our ankles etc. The point is we have to visualise the excess weight which we carry around on a daily basis.

So … what's your baggage allowance?

In addition, the things which are more important than your weight and waist measurements (to a great extent) are not quantitative, but rather qualitative. Here are the things which are important to have a look at:

Sleep!

Restless? Snoring? Waking up exhausted? These are major red flags for your overall health. Not to mention that your partner is probably annoyed by your snoring, earplugs in; or worse, genuinely worried because of the long asphyxiating pauses symptomatic of sleep apnoea. These are all indications that something needs doing, and doing now. Sleep apnoea is a condition that can increase your risk of heart attack and death! Snoring, more often than not, is caused by fat around your neck making it more common for your soft palate to collapse while sleeping as the jaw bone relaxes, thereby constricting your airway. Consequently you snore; and if the airway closes completely, you deprive your brain of oxygen until your brain jolts you awake to breath again like you just emerged from being held under the water in a bad dream.

So, flab is most likely the problem and if this is you, the importance sleep has on the way you feel and function can't be overstated. While we're at it... how old is your bed? And what's your pillow like? It may be time to nip down to Ikea and try a few out. A decent mattress is cheap in the scheme of things, or even a memory-foam chiropractic pillow is a cheap fix that can make a huge difference.

For me this moment came when I was uncomfortable in my clothes, and when I hit the scales after a long time of not bothering to check in with myself I was shocked to see 122Kg. I'd run out of holes on my straining belt. I was also feeling what I thought mistakenly was the aches and pains of AGE... But actually these aches and pains and ailments were the consequence of my poor physical condition. My neck and lower back were constantly seizing up and I was very uncomfortable. One major catalyst of change for me was my SNORING and this was a big warning flag. I was googling sleep clinics, and I was spending quite a bit of cash on physiotherapy appointments and massage therapists just to keep me feeling normal, not to mention being deluded that some gizmo would give me the sleep I knew I was missing.

Toxins

Let's talk about smoking, drinking, drugs and anything else that you know can be easily classified as a toxin – but let's be realistic. We are not monks, and we all have various bad habits that we will happily co-exist with. The point is to get real! No-one is telling you go give up that cigar or gin and tonic if that's your one vice and it helps keep you sane – but c'mon, you're not stupid … it's time to be objective. While we're at it, now is the time to have a proper look at your fridge and larder. Throw out the junk and don't buy it again (you can't consume it if it's not there – and to a large degree this journey begins in the supermarket).

Smoking

Even though, statistically speaking, 20% to 30% of all of us are likely to be smokers, I'm gonna come out and say it. While it seems like it's politically incorrect nowadays to point out that smoking is not all that smart health-wise (no judgement, of course), simply put, it causes death! It will kill you! Not today perhaps, but if you're engaging your common sense you know that it will carve about 20 years off your life expectancy, give or take a few years. More's the point, if it's going to take you out, it's not going to be pretty… heart attacks, cancer, emphysema and all of that! Not to mention that it's going to cost money – lots of it – and majorly screw up your breathing.

There no more basic function of being alive than breathing. So why compromise this most essential function… because it suppresses your appetite a bit? Calms your nerves? For women, if it does help you control your weight, no-one notices when you get to an age where your skin is sullen and crepe-like and your lips have micro-creases and you're sucking on a ciggy like a sailor – not a good look. Now, in light of Covid-19, the added risk of compromising your respiratory system is simply ridiculous when this is something that you have a say over.

Yes, it might give you a bit of a calm and it might be a habit you enjoy that provides a momentary time-out or a collegiate moment with your fellow smokers. Additionally, it is well known that nicotine is possibly one of the most addictive substances on Earth – but there are now patches, gums and other devices to help you quit. If you love your occasional cigar and that's your thing, then who is anyone to tell you not to indulge? But you have to ask yourself if you are willing to gamble 20 years of your life for that small pleasure. Of course smokers will point to Auntie 'so-and-so' who smoked like a chimney and because of her 'strong genes', to which you can claim some genetic relation, she went on to live to 103, etc. Not a great argument. So I invite you to be objective, as that's what we are being here. How much do you smoke? How does it make you feel? Do you want to change that? If so, you know you CAN do it. Of course you can, don't be ridiculous! You can do anything you put your mind to.

Caffeine

The world's most popular stimulant! I'm not saying you shouldn't have your tea or coffee either, but caffeine is a stimulant and strips your endocrine system and disrupts your sleep. If you are feeling anxious it could be your caffeine intake; it was for me. Count your coffees and teas. If you're having more than one or two a day, delete one, and replace it with something else (preferably broth). When established, repeat. Don't have caffeine after 2.00pm; or if you do, introduce decaf coffee or decaf tea! It's simple and you won't notice the difference. I like my coffee and tea (I was at 15 a day at one point!), so I'm down to a morning coffee and then I switch to one decaf in the evening. As you are reducing your caffeine intake, take a vitamin B complex (containing all the essential B vitamins) and before you know it you'll observe a big difference in your mood and sleep quality.

Drinking

This is going to be a tough one. Alcohol in its pure form is ethanol, a poison; but of course drinking is interwoven into our lives. I do believe that, as Jurgen Klopp, Liverpool FC's famous manager, said: "Sure we all enjoy a beer – but alcohol interferes with recovery, so why do it?" On the other hand, we are not athletes here and there are studies that purportedly report a positive correlation between small amounts of alcohol containing antioxidants such as those found in red wine (not the cheap shit you buy in the supermarket, but maybe an organic biodynamic example).

What's more important is the amount of sugar contained in beer, sugary alcoholic drinks and white wine (red wine has less sugar, generally speaking). Instead of thinking about a bottle of wine or a few beers, think of it as a big bottle of full sugar Coca-Cola! White wine and beer are high in carbohydrates, and additionally alcohol is metabolised as sugar – so it's much the same. All that sugar is keeping you out of ketosis and is going to make your journey very uphill. So, no-one said you have to stop drinking – but you can make changes and help yourself. For now, ask yourself how much you drink. Is it healthy, and actually… is it a problem for you to change?

From my experience, cleaner spirits work better (with diet mixers if need be); and I enjoy the odd red wine, assuming I can refrain from finishing the bottle!

Drugs

Drugs are a big subject and really we are talking about dependency. I once had an acquaintance who was a personal trainer who told me he regularly used cocaine. I was blown away by the contradiction that his body image could be so misaligned with his health. To be honest I'm not here to judge, and if you do drugs it's up to you; but ask yourself the question, and be honest with yourself.

I don't have any real experience with drug use apart from a few joints. However, we all need some escape, and much like drinking we like to banish our thoughts to oblivion. Yep – it's human, like I said. But firstly, are you smoking your drugs? In which case I refer back to what I said about smoking and your respiratory system. And secondly, if you have a problem giving up – then consider that you might have some dependency.

If you do, confront it head-on and resolve to do something about it as part of this little journey if it's gotten out of hand. Otherwise get some more serious professional help, starting with your doctor. But don't kid yourself that something you repeat 'every day' might not be a 'habit'. In fact it's worth really examining all the things we do 'every day', because they have a cumulative effect whether they are healthy or (more importantly) unhealthy.

Mental health

I'm listing mental health under possible toxins. In fact, mental health is possibly more important than all of the others combined if it leads to an open door policy to everything else and self-sabotaging behaviours generally. It's certainly a battle which everyone I know, including myself, has waged at times in their life; and it's great that this subject has become de-stigmatised in recent times.

So here are a few disturbing facts. Suicide is the leading cause of death in males between 18 and 40 in the UK, Australia and (I suspect) a whole swag of developed countries. Now, talking to the men out there, there's probably a whole book to be written on the effects of modern society on blokes – but I think a few things are clear. Being human, and more specifically being a bloke, in this day and age is tough. It's perhaps more complex than in past simpler times;

for most, the addition of job uncertainty, mortgages, children if you have them, plus the ceaseless flow of bills and financial commitments is reason enough. Not to mention the Covid-19 crisis and GFM (Global Financial Meltdown, as it's being described).

Add to the mix that, at this stage of life, health events begin to rear their ugly heads and that likely those around us start to fall prey to ill health and even death – whether it be parents or more worryingly those of our own generation. Anxiety and depression are rife and often not talked about between men; we just don't do it very well. Despite awareness, and campaigns to de-stigmatise the issue, men seem to internalise their issues and go with a 'suck it up' or 'fix it' attitude. It's a rock we push – as I heard it put – and we do it alone.

Mental health of course is not a uniquely male issue. For women, the post-childbirth years, career instability and relationship breakdown have equally toxic effects on wellbeing. Not to mention the menopause which can only be described as hormonal Armageddon. Plenty of women suffer from depression too, but women do this stuff a little better than men. When confronted by social issues, women naturally tend to support each other, call out for help, and give it freely.

In addition, societal norms tend to shame men into silence about the issues; and when you add isolation and shame to the mix it's a recipe for disaster.

So, there are a number of things which we need to borrow from the way women deal with mental health as a whole. If indeed equality is seen as a good thing, let's start by trying to have an equal life expectancy and address some of these disturbing stats.

Get a check-up!

If you haven't done so recently or are the type of person who won't go to the doctor unless you're at death's door … well, get to the doctor and have a general check-up, or 'wellness check' as it's commonly referred to. It will give you a baseline for any family history and blood markers prior to embarking on this journey. Remember that doctors can treat or manage almost anything if you catch it early enough! If you're a man, the old prostate needs a check too; and not to worry, if you don't fancy a finger up the bum they do it with a blood test these days.

If you are managing a severe illness or condition, obviously you need to consult your doctor and work with what you've got and within your limitations; but in the main, losing weight and adopting a healthier lifestyle will lower your reliance on medication and generally reduce the strain on your system. It makes sense. Don't use your ailments and conditions as an excuse, because we are talking about starting out by making small changes here. And everyone can make small changes.

It's not a bad idea to combine an overall check-up at the same time as taking your baseline measurements prior to starting. You will be able to track your progress as part of your tale of the tape – and your doctor can help you if needed.

CHAPTER 2

IT'S TIME TO START –
PLAN YOUR WORK, WORK YOUR PLAN

So you have an idea of where you are and where you want to be. But it's abstract in nature, a goal of perhaps your historical or imagined self – which to be honest, in all likelihood is not realistic. Brad Pitt and his six-pack again, or some equally impossible female equivalent.

Instead it is better to focus on your alternate self. This is the 'you' that you know is in there, hiding behind whatever has gotten in your way. It might be the version of you with more confidence, better self-esteem and more motivation. The only problem is that by the time you're rocking middle age, with the burdens of career and responsibilities of family life, for most it's easy to lose sight of that person.

Hence the mid-life crisis, post baby crash or meno-crisis happens for so many – when instead of addressing the issue, people seek to bridge the gap with knee-jerk life changes or material band-aids which are often self-destructive and are really just to distract ourselves from the larger questions we don't really want to confront. We cling to stories of ourselves which justify being rooted to the spot. Whether that be a physical condition or a social circumstance or even worse, blaming our bad genes! The old phrases: 'This won't work for me because I'm _____', or 'I try, I really do, but _____', usually get an airing right about now!

We witness a lurch (sometimes of desperation) and when others see it, everyone rolls their eyes as surely as if you'd just stuck a wig on your balding noggin, or pumped your face full of botox! So, what to do? Well there is a better version of you lurking back there … but a new car, paralysing your face, or some other band-aid isn't going to bring you closer to your ideal self, however tempting that might be.

It's better to visualise what the 'better' version of you looks like. Not the fantasy, but the possibility. If you have areas where you are lacking … which ones can you do something about? Can you fix your terrible teeth by a much-needed trip to the dentist? Do you need a haircut that is of this century? Does your fashion sense say old rather than young? Maybe; but what is certain is that for the vast majority of us, being overweight is easily the area which has the greatest impact on our health and self esteem. This can, and should, be the area most easily addressed.

The point is to identify what you can do something about, and what you can't. Some of it is superficial, and some of it is of a much deeper psychological nature.

So make a list of the things that your alternate self has, that you don't. Again this is not some fantasy … it is what you know deep inside that you should or could be. The laughable thing is that a good few of the items on your list will be so easy to remedy that you will know you are neglecting yourself when you articulate them. For what you cannot change, be stoic; and waste not an ounce of energy worrying about it.

Go to the doctor, have that check-up. Go to the dentist, have a check-up. Review your superficial appearance if you secretly know you are hiding your true self behind a facade or mask of some sort or a hairstyle from the '60s. Ask for the honest opinion of a few people who don't care about what you think (ask them not to hold back, and take note). This is not to say that you shouldn't accept yourself as God made you; but to look at what might be standing in the way of that.

As you lose weight and your self-image changes as fast as your waistline, review your clothes. If you have the same ill-fitting T-shirts, dresses, jumpers and trousers – maybe it's time to do a bit of shopping. Get with the times before you look like your grandparents did!

It's only when we visualise and articulate our alternate self that we define the differences between ourselves now and ourselves in the future. Again, it's not a bad exercise to write these down. On the basis of these visualisations, plans begin to formulate; and with those plans we can create micro-steps and micro-habits which move us in the right direction.

Simplicity

The key to doing anything that will last is making it simple. Simplicity in itself is, and should be, a goal – not just in the context of your health and nutrition but in all aspects of your life. If you can simplify something to make it easier, it creates less resistance to repeat and so forth. The over-complication of things is often what gets in the way of our achievements. Instead, the idea of breaking down things (like eating choices, exercise routines, etc) is to do simple things that are easy to repeat, and eliminate unnecessary complication.

For instance, making your exercise routine a fixed time of say 30 minutes, rather than a complicated gym session involving a lot of variables, is going to be more sustainable. Equally, a substitute for your weekly take-out pizza (you always order the same one, right?) with perhaps chicken drumsticks is the key to keeping it simple … chicken drumsticks replaces your favourite pizza, always. Then it's a no-brainer next time you come in late from work. Our brains are too lazy to compute complicated alternatives, especially when we are tired or hungry. Whatever is easy is a great answer when it's the healthiest choice! So pursue it as an end in itself.

Spark joy

There is a female Japanese tidiness guru by the name of Marie Kondo. If you haven't heard of her, she helps people clear their cluttered lives and saves their sanity in the process. It's quite fascinating how something so basic can have such a radical effect on everyday life.

Something she espouses is the concept of 'spark-joy'. To put it simply, if something doesn't spark some joy in you, it's time to dispense with it. She might be talking about your sock draw, but I'm talking about your life! Shitty job making you depressed? Time to rethink your career choices! Overweight? That's easily within your control. Toxic relationships that make you feel worthless? Time to confront the truth. Obligations weighing you down? Time to look at what you can cut to lighten the load!

These things are important, and if neglected they will put you in an early grave. You just need to identify them without attachment and make a plan to slowly but deliberately move in the right direction.

Attachment

My grandma once said, "Indifference is your greatest weapon." She was making a comment about some bully, but the application to life in general is useful. Developing a sense of detachment can make all the difference when viewing other people's judgement on what you are or what you are not; and formulating a plan which is right for you, without seeking permission.

In addition, indifference is different to an active position. It's easy to pretend you don't care when secretly you do, or take an opposing stance to something – because we are programmed to have reactions. However a reaction is not truly indifference. Indifference is a neutral position, which is neither engaged nor disengaged. It neither likes nor dislikes.

Why is this useful when we are transforming some aspect of our lives, such as weight loss? Because indifference to food, or people, or a job, is much less polarised than hating or loving something. Indifference is a calm sensation. It doesn't require your emotional or energetic involvement. It also severs your 'relationship' with something. You might be someone who 'loves' cupcakes or beer or whoever/whatever. If you feel like you are being asked or forced to quit or compromise on that thing or person, you will have a reaction. In all likelihood, that will be resistance. Resistance equals pain at some level – and so eventually you will return to your original position to alleviate that pain.

Indifference is 'letting go' so that it's easier to let go when you feel you are stuck. This will help with easing the rusty bolt that is getting in the way of you making headway in changing behaviours or attitudes which do not serve you well.

Mind your own business

As a child, odds are you've been told to mind your own business a few times.

However what does this really mean, or what can it mean? We are suffering an epidemic of 'over engagement' and 'over significance'. News, social media and everything else has resulted in us feeling lost and overwhelmed by the level of information we are expected to keep up with. Add to that work and professional matters, and now keep up with the plethora of bills, insurances and licences etc and that's it! Mentally, we're swamped. Transfixed by the chaos and rendered immobile by merely trying to keep up with factors that surround us. It's like we're hypnotised into a trance, and drawn ever deeper into the chaos.

So as an exercise, imagine that you have no sources of information at hand. No Internet, no news, no TV, no nothing; and now ask yourself how much of what happens in the world actually affects you and your daily life directly? Yeah, not much! Not much at all. Even in the Covid-19 pandemic it is worth remembering that millions of people will neither be affected, or know anyone who is affected, by something which is broadcast continually. This is not to take an unkind view of suffering … but unless we were told about something as worrisome as climate change, would it actually impact on our immediate life on a daily basis?

Extend that principle and ask yourself how much of what happens in your country, province, suburb, or even street, actually affects or has the slightest impact on your daily life. Yeah … still almost nothing! Although no-one is immune to economics. But even the train strike/store closure/neighbour's new fence etc, all, more than likely, have little or no actual effect on your life. Soon this approach may even seep into other aspects of your life and you will be able to 'tune out' the aspects over which you have no control, no interest, or no effect. It's the effect of more and more of us switching off the news. That's a good thing! Now, extend the principle.

The truth is that much of the time we feel a need for 'involvement' to be seen as valid. It feeds our egos. On a macro level we can be engaged in world issues, but really we have no impact on them so our views and actions are irrelevant. On a micro level too, you can be outraged at some local matter – but sticking your nose into it will likely not change a thing! Apart from putting you at odds with your community, locally or globally, and taking up your valuable energy, it will have no impact.

Now you're probably thinking that's probably a bit of a fatalistic view. Surely we can all contribute to change, and switching off to what's going on in the world is sticking our heads in the sand? That's true – BUT you can be a bit more discerning about what's your business and what's not. If you are putting these larger issues ahead of your own, particularly your own health, ultimately YOU are paying a very real price for this. It is also a handy way of procrastinating so as to not confront the real issues at hand.

Why is that relevant in the context of this book? Well again we are trying to establish what we can affect and what we can't, and furthermore we are not wasting our energy on the distractions of what is, in the grand scheme of things, none of our business. It is a different interpretation of the same theme of non-attachment.

I have long been a fan of saying 'none of my business' when asked my opinion. It also puts the boot on the other foot in the world of social media, where literally everything is (happily) none of my business – regardless of how much people try to make it so. To free yourself of the judgement and opinions of others, especially when it comes to what people will call a crazy way of eating, it is also useful to extend this concept to 'what you think of me, is none of my business'.

Learning to say no

Learning to say **NO** can be a lifelong lesson that is often never learned. It is possibly one of the most difficult and valuable lessons to learn in avoiding self-compromise in return for acceptance – whether that is seen as being nice, being expedient or just being agreeable. It has certainly been an issue for me in my life.

We are programmed in modern life to say YES. Yes to everything. Adopt a 'can do' attitude and aspire and achieve. As famed psychologist and author Dr Jordan B Peterson says, agreeableness is not associated with success!

However the word NO is a really uncomfortable word for most. It puts you in conflict. It places you at odds with those who ask things of you. People these days have become much more adept at asking for anything and everything – and if you don't place your hand up and say NO from time to time, you will surely have no time to do anything; much less focus on project 'me'!

NO is an uncomfortable habit, but like all micro-habits it's good to start small. When someone asks you for something small, just say no. It's not necessary to be rude or impolite, just be resolute in your response.

It could be as inconsequential as someone asking if you have the time. Just say no. Sorry. But you have a wristwatch on? Why are you being such a dick? Sure, but does owning a watch give someone the entitlement to require you to provide information that they could find for themselves by also wearing a watch, or looking at their phone? Of course this is trivial, but these are 'comfort exercises' designed to take us harmlessly out of our comfort zone. Now, in practice, nine times out of 10, I would just tell that person the time. But once in a while I say 'no, sorry, I can't help you'.

The more you say it, the slower the stream of questions becomes. It's not your duty to find the answer or solution to every question or problem that someone puts to you, and 'I don't know' or a simple but polite 'no' will set you free from the shackles of compliance.

Where's the remote? When does the milk expire? Has that report been handled? How do you do this? All these questions often are indirect or passive requests for action and they're asked because it's the easy way out – but ultimately it comes at your energetic expense.

Learn to identify a question as a disguised request. If you are brainwashed enough, you automatically respond to questions without even being asked. The truth is, you can't make space for yourself if you're making space for everyone else. So it's time to flex that muscle a little and get used to it. If you perceive yourself as a 'good' person, and likely agreeable, I assure you that you will not be naturally adept at this – but I suggest you work on it and prioritise yourself.

Don't decide – just choose

Procrastination is your enemy. It's often said that if we think about doing something for more than seven seconds, we will find a reason to avoid it; and our self-talk will quickly dissuade us from doing something that we may know is good for us, but inconvenient.

The trick is not to debate reasons leading to decisions, but to simply replace them with choices. A choice does not need a lengthy thought process, and it removes procrastination.

For instance, choose to go for a walk or run. Don't debate the reasons why you should or shouldn't. Once you get into the habit of choosing over debating decisions, I guarantee choosing food off a restaurant menu becomes a 10-second process. The unwanted side effect is that whoever you're with will seem very annoying with their incessant umm-ing and arr-ing as they ponder through every possible item on offer.

Keeping an open mind

Most people accept that change is not easy. In addition, we know that if we are resistant to new behaviours we will surely cement our old habits. In essence being closed-minded ensures the continuance of behaviour patterns which do not serve us well.

Put simply, being open allows us to entertain that there is room for improvement. Can you admit that simple fact? In our context, this manifests itself as being open-minded to a way of eating which frankly goes against the grain (no pun intended) of the plant-based eating fervour that is sweeping our planet, and to a lot of conventional thinking out there. This book is not meant to be plant-based or vegan-hating, but rather it is encouraging you to find your own sweet spot with a progressively ketogenic diet moving towards a carnivorous and zero carb way of eating … with an open mind.

If you start this or any process with a 'I could never do that, or I will always have to have my _____ etc' stance, then ask yourself if you're being too fixed in your attitudes. Are you allowing yourself the flexibility to be contributed to? If not, is this keeping you fat, unhealthy and unhappy?

CHAPTER 3

EAT YOURSELF HEALTHY –
AND SAY NO TO DIETING FOREVER!

The shortest diet book in the world comprises one sentence saying 'eat less and exercise more'. However it's not quite the case, is it? The reality is that a simple regime of eating less, and then enduring hunger, simply does not work. It's not necessarily a very pleasant experience either, and increasing evidence suggests that 'what we eat', and 'when we eat' are far more important that the number of calories consumed. If we are to sustain a new way of eating to maintain health and longevity, then we have to re-think the diet paradigm that we've all been sold for so long.

If you take away nothing else from this book, then take this one point on board: Dieting is a restrictive mindset which sets you up for failure from the outset. Even if you succeed you will invariably break/fail at some later stage because your mindset is positioned to see it as a binary 'succeed or fail' way of thinking. Instead, you have to adopt a 'nutrition'-based mindset, which is more akin to a lifestyle and which allows you to engage in a 'way of eating' which gives you a good routine that you can maintain easily.

It feeds you what you need, and allows you to heal. However, it's imperative that you drop the 'food as leisure', 'food as an answer to boredom' and 'food because of social expectation' attitudes. That doesn't mean that we can't eat tasty things, or go for dinner with friends, but this one aspect is the difference between people who are slim, trim and healthy all year round and those who lapse into being overweight and obese.

We also have to acknowledge that much of our western diet has been influenced by industry trying to persuade us to eat what is expedient and efficient to produce; not necessarily what is good for us. In addition big food companies are profit monsters, so no wonder we are being encouraged to eat ALL the time. We now live in a feeding frenzy, and our health in the developed world has never been worse. Famously, in 1894, John Harvey Kellogg developed cornflakes as a bland morning meal as part of his extreme diet – promoted by his church – aimed at supressing masturbation! I'm serious … Google it!

What we eat and when we eat is much more important than exercise in achieving a weight loss goal, and increasingly in averting a lot of diet-induced dysfunction and ill health. The simple fact is that white refined carbohydrates and processed foods with high levels of refined sugars are playing havoc with your system. Generally, the 80/20 proportion fits pretty well, with nutrition contributing about 80% of the picture and allowing 20% for exercise. We have to remember that if health is the ultimate goal, we are wanting to lose body fat and gain some lean body mass in the form of muscle. Interestingly this doesn't have to involve hours and hours of laborious cardio, but we do have to get active! There is just no getting away from it.

The trick is that, when you are active, as you will have experienced, it motivates you to eat better – releasing feel-good chemicals that make you feel great. Consequently, once you are eating better and feeling lighter, you are more inclined to continue being more active. It's a virtuous circle, and therefore exercise is useful and essential; but what's going to give you immediate results is micro-habiting and redirecting the way you eat rather than going on a calorie-restrictive diet and killing yourself and your wallet with a gym membership!

First things first. We will one by one attack the big five offenders that you can count on your hand – and honestly this alone will get you some great results.

– **BREAD**
– **RICE**
– **PASTA**
– **ROOT VEGETABLES**
– **SUGAR, including sugar-laden/high carb Alcohols (and let's add Processed Foods in there as an extra)**

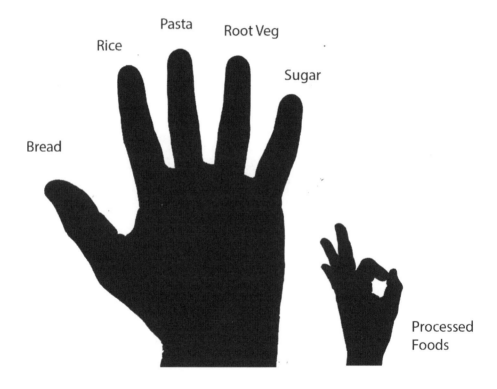

Seeing as these staples form the foundation of most of what we eat on a standard western diet, it's important to ease into it and attack the biggest offender for you personally. You'll know instantly which one is the issue for you. Are you the bread monster, or do you have a bottle of Chardonnay every night? Or do you have your six-pack of beer without even blinking? Just because you don't have a problem with rice, for instance, it doesn't mean you're not seriously connected to one of the others which is tanking your health and weight-loss efforts.

All of these foods metabolise as sugars, which if not used for immediate energy (for example, during exercise) are stored as fat. They spike your insulin – and because four of the five are refined, they do it very fast. Generally they are terrible low quality foods from a nutritional standpoint! In addition, the grains cause an inflammatory response.

Redirect your habits

A simple approach to redirecting your habits which works without fail is to just do two things. The first is to swap out something. Make a rule that one thing replaces the other and that's it. As mentioned previously, chicken replaces pizza, salad replaces pasta, or sparkling water replaces wine. Whatever… make your replacement strategy and stick to it. Once it's a habit and 'you don't mind it' extend the principle and replace something else. That's the HOW. It's pretty straightforward and pretty painless. If you're telling me you can't swap out pizza for chicken wings then you're not trying very hard.

Now we're going to cover the following basic strategies – which can be used alone or in conjunction to compound the results. The objective is to make things as easy and convenient as possible.

They are:

– **Progressive elimination of foods until you are zero-carb or close to it, and you have a high quality, nutrient-dense, predominantly carnivorous diet.**
– **Intermittent and therapeutic fasting, starting with only eating when you're hungry.**

Basic elimination

Elimination diets go from 'vegan' at one end through to 'carnivore' at the other, and the myriad in between. The problem is that if you go digging, you will find science, evidence and champions to support each and every approach, and the many variations in between, as well as to vilify the opposite end of the spectrum.

Plant-based proponents will point out the evils of meat consumption and vice-versa. So how do you choose? Given that we are individuals, please yourself. And as the carnivore pioneer Dr Shawn Baker wisely said: "Treat yourself as a sample of one in your own private eating and health experiment."

It may sound counter-intuitive, but science and following the evidence-based doctrine is somewhat subjective. People will say 'this is science, this is evidence-based, and whatever you're doing is crazy'. The problem however is that nowadays we can find evidence to support anything if we go looking for it, and plenty of peer groups to support it, and then build a case around what we think and want to justify. We only have to look at any hot political subject debate to show that science, to some degree, has become subjective … or at the very least selective.

I urge you to draw your own conclusions and find your own path and not to judge others' choices. There are people who (seem to) thrive on a plant-based diet, and those who have equally amazing results from eating only red meat, salt and water. Both extremes, it has to be said, have adopted versions of eating which, more often than not, have cut out the main offenders, and combined that solution with a rigorous exercise regime. So don't judge. This book is about pointing out things to be aware of, as well as some personal insight, without getting too judgy. However the motivation for this book is from the many friends who asked 'talk me through it' when losing a stack of weight and achieving healthy blood-work for the first time in 20 years and maintaining it over a prolonged period of time.

So, yes, if you want to be a vegan who also cuts out the big five (bread, rice, pasta, root vegetables, sugar and processed foods) – some benefits are common to both approaches. However beyond that, this book focuses more on a low carbohydrate approach and the benefits of eating meat!

If you feel you are suffering because of your reactions to certain foods, an elimination approach takes you back to a 'simplified' diet to get to the bottom of your issues. Elimination diets work because they take you back to scratch – but you have to do this slowly to avoid toxicity dumping, and strong reactions to foods you have become reliant on.

So what's the problem with Veg anyway?

Before we talk about vegetables, let's talk about grains. They have been sold to us over the years and they are singularly responsible for the large majority of havoc in our diet. We don't digest them well, they cause inflammation, and when refined they do horrible things to our insulin. So forget all that heart-smart multi-grain bread and cereal nonsense. That stuff is literally killing you, and plenty of other people. Gluten intolerance is now well known, but that's just the start of it.

We've all been told that the nutrients and fibre in vegies will be the cure-all in providing a balanced diet. Of course plants have some protein and some of the trace minerals that meat provides, but you also have to eat truckloads of them to compete with the nutritional density and values of meat, fish and poultry; and even moreso red meat. In addition your digestive system has a lot of fibre to deal with and frankly there are plenty of unwanted side effects to your gut once you start loading up on large quantities of vegetables.

Blood sugar and carbohydrate regulation can be hard to maintain, resulting in energy peaks and troughs – as anyone who has felt themself 'fading' at work after a carb-laden lunch can attest.

Also there is something called oxalates to consider and other substances, which come under the banner of 'anti-nutrients'. Oxalic acid is a toxic substance that vegetables produce in varying quantities as a kind of natural pesticide. Oxalates bind with calcium and form kidney stones and are highly toxic and actually block absorption of nutrients. Before adopting a plant-based diet, make sure you research these to avoid possible reactions to your health concerns. So just because it's green that doesn't necessarily mean it's good. We've all been getting 'sold' on the concept that anything plant-based is good to a certain degree. Now, these things may not be a big issue for you personally (they are not for me); but if you have sensitivities, these can become quite pronounced.

For instance, lets take spinach as a very typical example. It is very high in iron, right? We all know that. Popeye's favourite food! Maybe the first advertised 'super-food'. However, on its own we have difficulty metabolising it! Iron from food comes in two forms: Heme and non-heme. Heme is found only in animal flesh like meat, poultry and seafood. Non-heme iron is found in plant foods like whole grains, nuts, seeds, legumes and leafy greens. The form of iron found in spinach is non-heme which is generally poorly absorbed in the gut compared to heme iron from animal sources.

Secondly, spinach has extremely high levels of oxalic acid. This acid, again naturally present in vegetables, binds with iron which blocks its absorption in the gut.

We can reduce this effect to some degree by cooking spinach, but nowadays raw spinach salads are pretty common as when it's used as a lettuce alternative; and then juicing probably just super-concentrates the issue and in my view could be quite toxic.

So are these 'super-foods' doing more harm than good? This is not a class in spinach, but a demonstration that many 'healthy' foods can be anything but healthy. Do your own research and see what happens to things like wheat-grass in the gut, or what happened to Ashton Kutcher when he adopted Steve Jobs' fruitarian diet (he was hospitalised, if you were wondering), or indeed what happened to Liam Hemsworth when he went vegan.

A 'so-called' balanced diet

For most of us, an omnivorous approach seems to make sense. Eat everything in moderation; and by adding some animal protein, you end up at a stereotypical view of 'eating healthy' … fresh fruit and vegetables, whole grains, healthy oils, nuts, seeds and some animal protein, usually in moderate amounts. The old food pyramid including five a day, foods of different colours, etc, must surely be the safest way to avoid a nutritional gap. But is it?

The truth is that unless you are 'very good' and start adopting some restriction, this approach of 'eat a bit of everything' transitions into an attitude of 'eat a bit of anything and everything' and encourages poor self-regulation.

Additionally as we fall into an 'eat a bit less' mindset we find ourselves at the beginning of a restrictive calories-in calories-out mindset and the hunger highway quickly follows.

The problem that any so-called balanced diets run into is combining sugars and fats. You don't quite use all the sugars from carbohydrates for energy, as most of us lead a sedentary lifestyle … especially as we get older. So unless you are severely restricting and regulating your intake, that excess sugar turns to stored fat; and congratulations, you now have a gut!

We will eat healthy for a bit, until we don't. It's not different enough to have an effect, and doesn't short-circuit how our bodies process energy to eliminate excess weight and maintain it in the long term. So we have to challenge this conventional wisdom.

Hunger!

Inevitably you want to get to a point where you are only eating when you start feeling hungry, or 'peckish'. Peckish is the feeling you want to get friendly with. It's not hunger, but it's a cue that you want or need to eat. If you can get comfortable with waiting for that one cue alone, and not eating until that cue, then that's all you have to do! Don't eat until you feel hungry. Deceptively simple, and surprisingly hard.

If we don't eat until our bodies give us that signal then we are achieving quite a few things, which give us the tool kit to move forward. You don't have to feel hungry on this way of eating, but you do have to wait until your body gives you that signal to eat. For many people they simply have never had to wait. So if you're **not** hungry at 9.00am, 1.00pm or whenever you have traditionally eaten breakfast, lunch or dinner … just wait until you are. Hunger is a hormone called Ghrelin, and research shows it's an essential player in all sorts of long-term health benefits. So if we never even allow our bodies to signal when to eat, we might be inadvertently depriving ourselves of a whole host of essential positive side effects.

Firstly, by increments, minutely at first, we are shrinking our stomachs. Literally! Just as in the same manner as when we overeat, we are stretching our stomachs. A doctor friend told me that the feeling when we feel stuffed is actually our stomach bruising from being stretched to accommodate more food than it needs. Yuck! Kinda gross!

If you can acknowledge that your current eating habits are social rather than driven by your body's requirement to eat, then you are halfway there. So instead of eating when you are expected to, only eat when you are hungry; and more importantly, stop eating when you are not. That is literally the other half of the battle. You will get comfortable with the feeling you can start bringing in a bit of routine with this, and at that point you're halfway to fasting anyway – but see Chapter 4 for more on that.

Hunger vs. Thirst

We are always being advised to drink copious amounts of water. However, there is a reason that we have a sense of 'thirst' and that is why it is a natural trigger to hydrate and drink some fluids. What is important is not to confuse thirst with hunger. Often hunger and thirst kind of overlap, so keeping properly hydrated means that hunger is kept at bay.

Generally speaking it's not a bad idea to start and finish the day with a good-sized glass of water. This allows the body to flush toxins etc, including ketones, and helps with any immediate feelings of hunger. You will be surprised that as long as you are drinking water or broth of some kind, the 'hunger' for food seems to curiously evaporate.

Ditch Milk!

If you are sensitive to dairy, ditch milk altogether.

You may have already done this in order to achieve ketosis. Milk comprises big fat proteins, which is sugar in the form of lactose. Anyone who is lactose intolerant will tell you the effect on the gut!

Interestingly when milk is transformed to cheese and yogurt etc, the fermentation process changes the protein structure – which makes it much different to 'milk'. So if you want to stay fat … drink milk.

For me personally and many others when eliminating dairy, many report (me included) a great improvement in mental clarity and focus, and a huge reduction in mucus production and improvement in sinus health. This has become highly relevant in the Covid-19 discussion, as foods that promote mucus production do not help in ear, nose and throat conditions when fighting a respiratory disease.

You may choose to reintroduce cheeses, as I have, with virtually none of the effects that milk brings on. Again, experiment to see what's right for you.

What about Atkins/Paleo? Isn't it all the same?

They all have a lot in common in that they work on the same basic principle which is elimination, and low carbohydrates resulting in ketosis; however these specific diets taken in isolation introduce the mindset of restriction and rules and so it's difficult to climb back on the wagon it you stray. Also what seems to be a missing component is the concept of a slow transition. Going from an appropriately named SAD diet (Standard American Diet) to any zero carb plan often results in feeling terrible, which is often referred to as Keto Flu!

Also a word of caution: Relying on ketone production is not for everyone. Some people have metabolic disorders that make it impossible for their bodies to use ketones as fuel, so they must eat carbohydrates to live (this is a very, very small percentage of people). Other people take certain medications, carry certain genes, or have kidney issues that can all make ketogenic-based eating dangerous for their health. Anyone thinking about trying this with a stack of health issues should consult a doctor. However nutritionists and doctors generally agree that nobody's system should run on sugar and carbs alone. So, unless you are in that medically defined group, simply stating 'I can't function without my carbs' is just an excuse.

Transitioning slowly by initially eating healthier carbs such as cauliflower, avocado, nuts etc to divert yourself from going back to the big five is a good idea. When you do this you may start falling out of ketosis (or get close to it). Who cares? You have changed the habit and the main thing is that you are no longer hungry and you are filling up with 'better' stuff, not the bad stuff. Over time, you might be having some carbs which will make your keto levels dip, but not enough to bust out of ketosis altogether. Some (disciplined) people do this all the time and it's sometimes called 'keto-surfing', but again this defeats the main purpose – which is an easy to follow, easy to maintain approach.

With time, the goal is to start eating more nutrient-dense food (i.e. meat), and only eating when you are hungry. Meat is higher on the satiety scale (as are things like eggs) meaning it keeps you feeling fuller for longer. Soon you'll be craving steak instead of that big plate of veg, and eggs and bacon will once again become a guilt-free option.

The problem with starches is that they are high on the glycaemic index. What that means is that they give you energy very fast and are absorbed by your bloodstream extremely quickly. That's why athletes will usually load up on pasta or bread if they intend to do some vigorous activity where they need to increase their energy. But if you don't use that energy, guess what it turns into: Fat.

If you're having that pasta for dinner with a creamy sauce, the packet of corn chips or biscuits with a milky drink before bedtime, that's going nowhere but onto your waistline.

So what should we do about these food items, which form the basis of almost every dish you can think of? The problem is that commercially these ingredients are cheap, and they offer no nutritional value. So when you go to a food hall, cafe or restaurant, these are the items that they are trying to sell you or give you first so that you fill up on cheap useless stuff – instead of having to be fed more expensive, more nutritious ingredients.

Once you spot this, you see it everywhere; and if you're trying to avoid bread, rice and pasta then you realise how much of it is being literally forced down your throat and how convenience has largely got you to the state that you're in.

It goes without saying that your food choices start in the supermarket. Don't buy the bread to start with and make sure you buy non-carb replacements. For pasta and rice, I simply replaced them with Cos lettuce hearts to start off with. If it grows above the ground it is generally a leafy green of some sort. Nowadays almost all supermarkets sell bags of salad that are washed and ready to eat, which makes it very easy, and really if you're not taking advantage of this convenience, then you should. Although we will eventually move to reduce carbs even further, having a bag of washed salad is ultimately far superior to a bag of chips or a bowl of rice. For quite some time I continued with this strategy with good steady results.

Before we talk about sugar generally, let's talk about fruit. To be perfectly honest with you although people go on about fruit being high in sugar I think that fruit generally speaking is something that we would eat in the normal course of foraging. However it is highly unlikely that we would have fruits available year round at the point of being ripe. It's simply not a food source that we would have a lot of access to. If you think of yourself as a forager at heart, rather than a farmer, you might eat the amount of fruit that we would normally have in our diet.

However as you transition into a very low-carb environment, you will find that you become adapted to fat as your main energy source ('fat-fuelled' as it has become known). Once you are adapted, fruit does not do wonders for your stomach. For berries equally these would be seasonal, occasional and small in quantity. The same should be the case when consuming most fruits – and again, think of fruit as 'candy bombs' which will put you back out of ketosis and delay your weight loss trajectory and more than likely play havoc with your guts as mentioned. I recently had a bowl of strawberries and cream … I don't mind telling you that I paid the price for it (think bloating, stomach cramps and diarrhoea) all evening long. This is what I mean by pretty soon your low-carb lifestyle will become your new normal, because I couldn't wait to get back to my usual way of eating. This way of eating is littered with many 'okay, won't be doing that again' moments!

Sugar

The white death, they call it! Sugar is in almost everything, but especially processed food. Often disguised in what you think might be a healthy dish or plain ingredient jar of sauce, if it's been manufactured by a company it will usually have considerable levels of seasonings, stabilisers and (of course) sugars in it. What that means is that quite often you are consuming incredible amounts of sugar without even realising it. On closer examination when you look at the sugar content of an average can of soft drink, you realise that there are up to 32 grams of sugar in a can of full-sugar cola or any other soft drink. When a teaspoon of sugar weighs four grams you realise that there are six to eight teaspoons of sugar in every can; 24 spoons of sugar in a one-litre bottle, and 48 spoons in a two-litre (half gallon) bottle … 48 spoons! As an exercise, get a bag of sugar out and measure that quantity – it's shocking to see!

Now of course most people are aware of this and that's why zero-sugar soft drinks etc are quite popular.

But what about when you enjoy a gin and tonic, or a Red Bull and vodka, and (generally) other mixers that go with alcohol – especially in pubs, clubs, bars and restaurants when diet mixers are often not available? They are all very high in sugar and if you're a drinker, you're consuming much more sugar than you are alcohol. If you're on beer or wine, you might as well be drinking full-sugar soft drinks.

Now I confess I have a sweet tooth and could easily down a bar of chocolate or a packet of sweets. However once you've decided that you're gonna try and cut sugar out, you have to be a little bit more diligent about doing so beyond the obvious. One of the first steps is to read the label. It is incredible the amount of things that contain hidden sugar, and even (recently) sugar-free confectionery can contain high levels of carbohydrate. Quite often it's equally the savoury foods which contain base sugars (disguised as high fructose corn syrup) to 'improve' the flavour of sauces; not to mention all the other varieties of chemicals, etc.

Alcohol

As previously mentioned in the toxins section, dodge beer and white wine and full-sugar mixers. Swap these out for white spirits or even whiskey – which tend to be a lot lower in sugar than other drinks. Additionally, switch out your white wine and get in touch with your red wine self and have a glass of red instead of a bottle of white.

If we take the gradual approach, and we start to reduce the amount we are drinking by one or two over a period of time and then swap out the types of drinks that we are having, then the impact to our blood sugar and liver is probably not an issue. However alcohol contributes a lot of 'wasted' calories and although we are not counting them, they will stack up to slow our journey. That said, I'm sitting here with a fat glass of bourbon … so find your own pace that works for you. Cheers!

If you are serious about getting a flat stomach, cutting out alcohol altogether will eliminate a lot of excess calories – but you have to take into account the social element that alcohol plays in our lives. You also have to be honest with yourself.

Sweets and Candy

For those of us with a sweet tooth, sugars of the more common variety such as sweets, candy, lollies, chocolate bars etc are a tough nut to crack. You can gradually reduce these until they are out altogether while re-educating your palate. I started by swapping out sweets with some kind of coated nuts like honey cashew nuts etc and then I went down to the savoury varieties of those things including almonds and cashew nuts.

As for chocolate, I knew that this was going to be difficult. I started swapping out milk chocolate for dark chocolate, and then only having >80% cocoa – again looking at the carb content for each. This means you can have a few squares of chocolate with a coffee and not feel like you are being deprived. After a few months, instead of Maltesers, I was snacking on some salted cashews; and instead of a big bar of Cadbury's, I'd have a few squares of dark chocolate.

I even take a small bag of snacks to the movie theatre (cashews/beef jerky and a few squares of dark chocolate or whatever) so that I don't get drawn into a bag of sweets or popcorn, which is easy to do. Again, it's quantity. I've now stopped my little cashew nut addiction because when I give myself permission to eat them I tend to eat a whole bag. Not dreadful in the scheme of things, but they will bump me out of ketosis; and now I'll take some beef jerky if I have it.

If you just need the odd sweet from time to time, of course there are more and more sugar-free ones out there. But check the carbohydrate value in them and beware that many can have a laxative effect and cause painful gas. At least the ones from Aldi did!

Soft drinks and artificial sweeteners

While we are talking about the movie theatre, another thought about soft drinks. Artificial sweeteners, in the past, were usually saccharine-based. Saccharine/aspartame is toxic and is a known carcinogen (how on Earth is it even allowed on the shelves?) however Xylatol and other sugar-derived sweeteners have been around for a while and now we are starting to see much healthier alternatives like Stevia etc. Most of the soft drinks that we can see nowadays contain phenylalanine, sucralose or something similar. Now while these may not be good for you, they are a damn site less harmful to your waistline than sugar. So if you have a sweet tooth, diet drinks might be poison; but for my purposes, they are a way to feel that you are having something that tastes sweet without affecting your waistline or triggering your insulin response in the same way that refined sugar does.

CHAPTER 4

THERAPEUTIC AND INTERMITTENT FASTING

This topic deserves a book all of its own, and indeed there are many. In my view it is as important as what you eat, in managing your weight loss; if not moreso in boosting all sorts of hidden health benefits; so before you skip this chapter and think fasting is synonymous with going hungry, please read on because you'd be wrong!

So what is fasting? Basically it's not eating … **but,** that doesn't mean you necessarily go hungry because with this type of fasting, you keep your hunger at bay by drinking **BROTH**. Broth in fact will mean you never really feel hungry at all, and in addition you get an amazing nutrient-dense concoction that frankly will do wonders for your health. More on broth later.

Intermittent fasting has long been used as a hack by body builders to lose fat quickly while maintaining lean muscle mass. What underpins it is a much more ancient and well founded approach to maintaining health and hacking your metabolism. In fact it's a mainstay of almost every mainstream religious philosophy and cultural tradition, but somehow in the last 100 years or so it has been forgotten and ignored, and it has to be noted this has happened in direct relation to the unprecedented rise of obesity and ill health.

It's also become something of a modern day 'no-brainer' as we all adapt to trying to deal with the ever-increasing complexity of eating routines and the busy lives we lead. However, fasting is so deceptively simple that when we commit to eating within a reduced time window, the benefits are progressive, compounding and cumulative.

Here are the five stages of fasting:

1. **Ketosis leading to heavy ketosis** after 12 and 18 hours
2. **Autophagy** after 24 hours
3. **Growth hormone production** after 48 hours
4. **Insulin reduction** after 54 hours
5. **Immune stem cell rejuvenation** after 72 hours

Love

Now, if you're like me, you've read that and gone: What? 72 hours! Dude, that's three days without food… are you mental? However like everything else this is something that you should ease into. I should mention that I've never done anything beyond a 48-hour fast, but I plan to experiment in my own sweet time. I think half of it is psychological; in fact I know it is. Extended fasting is not a pre-requisite to losing weight it should be said, but fasting intermittently until you can feel comfortable eating once or twice a day, without snacking, probably is.

Anyway, the first step would be to start by cutting out snacking, so you can have a solid 12 hours between dinner and the next day's breakfast (literally break-fast). Eventually you can contain your eating to an 18-hour window by either cutting out breakfast or having an early dinner. In time, with the help of sufficient electrolytes (i.e. salty broth) and hydration, you might be ready for OMAD (one meal a day); and then venture into trying a longer fast periodically.

So let's go through what happens in the stages of fasting, one at a time:

1. Ketosis and heavy ketosis

Ketosis as the name suggests is what's behind the, now ever-increasingly popular, ketogenic diet. It is a metabolic state when you have exhausted glucose as an energy source and instead are starting to use fat as an energy source. This usually occurs after

12 hours of fasting. Your liver secretes ketones in this state, and it is measurable by the amount of acetone secreted in your urine or breath. You can test for this with urine analysis strips from the chemist; or a breath sensor, which works much like a breathalyser. I can recommend one called the KETOSTICK, which comes with a handy app to keep track of your process – but there are many others out there, including some that measure your glucose levels too.

The state of ketosis builds gradually, so when you reach heavy ketosis, you are using fat almost exclusively as an energy source – not least by your brain. This ketone usage by your brain is one of the reasons that fasting is often claimed to promote mental clarity and positive mood – ketones produce less inflammatory products as they are being metabolised, than does glucose; and they can even kick-start production of the brain growth factor BDNF!

After the 18-hour mark of fasting, you're in deep fat-burning mode or heavy ketosis and are generating significant ketones. Ketones are important because they can act as signalling molecules, similar to hormones, to tell your body to activate stress-busting pathways that reduce inflammation and repair damaged DNA. Interestingly the ketogenic diet was developed as a way to manage epilepsy – which should tell you all you need to know about the inflammatory effects of a diet high in refined white carbohydrates and grains on your brain function.

2. Autophagy

Within 24 hours, your cells are switching into another gear. As we progressively starve our cells of nutrition they turn away from 'growth mode' and turn to processes that look to efficiency. Autophagy literally means self-eating, and the body recycles and eliminates things like folded proteins. In this state genes are triggered which are related to fat metabolism, stress resistance and damage repair. High levels of ketone bodies appear to reactivate these genes – leading to reduced inflammation and stress resistance in the brain, for example.

When your cells can't, or don't, initiate autophagy, bad things happen – including neuro-degenerative diseases. Autophagy is an important process for cellular and tissue rejuvenation because it removes damaged cellular components including mis-folded proteins linked to things like Alzheimer's and other neuro-degenerative diseases.

3. Growth hormone production

Part of the ageing process, as we know it, is linked to a drop in human growth hormone. It is why our metabolism slows, we lose muscle mass, our hair falls out, we lose elasticity in our skin and lots of other not-so-fun stuff. Hence the lack of human growth hormone for the 50-and-over age group is a big problem regarding inflammation issues, and breakdown of joint mobility etc.

I'm not suggesting taking it as a supplement because we have the ability to generate it naturally through fasting, and frankly taking hormones is a dangerous business. However if we can stimulate it naturally, growth hormone helps preserve lean muscle mass and reduces fat accumulation – particularly as we age. It also appears to play a role in longevity and can promote wound healing and heart health – so it cannot be overstated in terms of its importance for middle age, and delaying the onset of conditions associated with old age.

By 48 hours without calories or with very few calories, carbs or protein, ketone bodies produced during fasting increase your growth hormone level up to five times as high as when you started your fast. Ghrelin, the hunger hormone, also promotes growth hormone.

So although we don't want to introduce hunger as a part of the program, experiencing it or getting to the point where we are comfortable with it can have its benefits.

4. Insulin reduction

At the 54-hour mark, your insulin has dropped to its lowest level point since you started fasting, and your body is becoming increasingly insulin-sensitive which is a good thing.

Lowering your insulin levels has a range of health benefits both short-term and long-term. Lowered insulin levels put a brake on the insulin and mTOR (see following) signalling pathways, activating autophagy. Lowered insulin levels can reduce inflammation, make you more insulin sensitive (and/or less insulin resistant, which is especially a good thing if you have a high risk of developing diabetes). If you are diabetic or pre-diabetic this should be reason enough to explore this further. It also protects you from chronic diseases of ageing, including cancer.

Studies in mice have shown that prolonged fasting (greater than 48 hours) leads to stress resistance, self-renewal and regeneration of blood cell stem cells. Through this same mechanism, prolonged fasting for 72 hours has been shown to preserve healthy white blood cell or lymphocyte counts in patients undergoing chemotherapy, which takes us on to…

5. Immune STEM cell rejuvenation

In a well-fed state, the individual cell in your body is in 'growth' mode. Its insulin and other signalling functions tell the cell to grow, divide and synthesise. By the way, these signals, when overactive, have implications in cancer growth as you would expect. So could a clue to beating cancer lie in simply starving cells of nutrition periodically? Quite possibly. It certainly makes common sense to me that an over-fed cell would be more inclined to proliferate, where as a cell periodically starved of its signals to divide might behave differently.

The 'mammalian target of rapamycin' or mTOR, is one of these signal pathways and loves having plentiful nutrients around – especially carbohydrates and proteins. When active, mTOR tells the cell not to bother with autophagy as already mentioned. The well-fed cell isn't worried about being efficient and recycling its components – it's too busy growing and dividing.

What you really need to know is that the well-fed cell has many genes signals turned on, including those associated with cellular survival and proliferation.

In a well-fed state, your cells turn on those signals; but they also turn other genes' signals off. These include genes related to fat metabolism, stress resistance and damage repair. Actually, when you fast, some of those ketone bodies appear to reactivate these genes, leading to lowered inflammation and stress resistance.

Bonus stage: Refeeding!

We nearly forgot about the last and perhaps most important stage of fasting – the refeeding stage! It's important to break your fast with something light but nutritious, that will further improve the function of cells and tissues that went through clean-up while you were fasting. Simple foods are best, and as always stay away from carbs and sugars which, while tempting, may in fact lead to problematic blood sugar spikes. I tend to break a fast with a cup of broth, and some chicken or fish … something light. Although steak is always on the menu! Even so, I start with small amounts rather than a giant serving.

Now in practice, like everything, people who fast can take it on as a bit of an endurance sport. I'm not suggesting you go into prolonged fasting straight off, or without medical consultation. However, start small and see how you go. Many of the benefits for our purposes can be achieved doing a 24-hour fast, or intermittently fasting 23 hours and eating in a one-hour window. This essentially becomes the OMAD or one meal a day way of eating. And it is an easy routine to keep to. In my experience it can become quite addictive in its simplicity and routine.

Once a week or month, or what ever works for you, introduce a longer fast for the above stated reasons. Go for it. I currently eat within a one- or two-hour window, usually dinner time; and more recently have loosely started skipping eating on one day of the week, in my case Mondays or Wednesdays, as they fit my schedule!

So how do you manage to not get hungry during the 23 hours or more, and what constitutes a fast? The answer is …

BROTH

This might be a chapter on its own as it has so many benefits, but I think it sits well in the fasting section because it's what allows you to fast comfortably for as long as you like while filling your belly and feeding your soul.

Broth comes in many shapes and sizes and is as varied as there are people and cultures. From chicken soup referred to as the Jewish Penicillin, to the beef bone broth which I'm going to suggest, they all are essentially the same base ... bones plus salt plus water, plus maybe a few herbs and spices!

Regardless of the animal, chicken, beef, pork etc, the bones have incredible levels of nutrients in them. They have cartilage, marrow and the bone itself. The addition of salt is essential as it draws out all these nutrients.

Cartilage turns to collagen; bones release their calcium, magnesium and hundreds of other trace minerals. Ladies, if you think that putting some cream on your face is going to make your skin look younger, then you will save a fortune when you treat your skin from the inside out. Your hair will never look better and frankly you will feel a million bucks when you make broth a part of your life.

Now in terms of micro-habits, it's easy to replace tea and coffee with a cup of broth – although there is nothing to stop you enjoying a coffee in the morning. I sometimes add a spoon of mustard, some garlic and dried herbs, but that's just me. I also tend to gravitate to beef bones and I get these from the butcher. I just ask for some bones for the dog, and it depends on your butcher as to whether he charges for them or not. Either way they are CHEAP. Chicken frames, or any other bones will do. Salted pork bones make super-tasty broth!

The broth also contains some essential fats to keep your energy up, and yourself energised, but one of the most important ingredients in the broth is the salt. The salt or sodium component keeps our electrolytes up. Without it we feel light-headed, devoid of energy and frankly our muscles don't function well and will eventually cramp up in a low-salt environment (which is why all those sports drinks are essentially sweetened salt replacement drinks).

> I GUARANTEE you, if when you start to feel peckish or hungry, you have a cup of bone broth ... you will soon be on one meal a day (OMAD).

To transition into fasting, forget the old adage that breakfast is the most important meal of the day – because the slogan was likely developed by a cereal-marketing department. The best way is to simply skip breakfast. By doing this you will have cut your food intake by 25% to 30% and extended your fasting window from nine or 10 hours to 14 or 15 hours.

If you have a late lunch or early dinner you easily fall into the 16 and eight pattern (16 hours fasted and feeding within an eight-hour window).

So the side benefits are quite obvious (but a surprise nonetheless): It's a lot cheaper! You don't have to worry about food choices, preparation and clearing up etc. It starts to simplify your life drastically. Pretty soon you will witness the constant feeding frenzy and associated mania of those around you, especially if you work. You will save a fortune on worktime lunches, or packing a lunch; but then at the same time you will realise how much of our eating is purely social convention. My reply to 'shall we get something to eat' is 'sure, I'll come and watch you eat', as I have now developed an ease with my own way of eating. And no doubt you will too.

I generally replace lunch with a cup of broth or two, but obviously it's not always practical to have a slow-cooked home-made broth available. I use a Thermos flask, and nowadays the insulated steel drink bottles are ideal. Additionally there are some commercial bone broth concentrates available which contain grass-fed beef, water and salt boiled down to a thick concentrate the texture of honey. They are a little pricey but they last 'ages' and in the scheme of things are very convenient. Unfortunately products like Bovril etc are mainly yeast extract even though they purport to be beef extract, and they fall into the processed category. Shame! However, the one I use is called 'Best of the Bone' and it comes from 100% grass-fed Australian cattle and contains nothing but the concentrated extract of bones, salt and water.

In Broth we trust!

The Bulletproof coffee and MCT oil

Like many of us, I like my coffee and have it with Stevia sweetener and a little heavy pouring cream; however I started reading about people raving about the Bulletproof Coffee and putting butter and MCT Oil in their coffee. What the hell? I did my own research about MCT Oil.

MCT Oil is a supplement often added to smoothies, the so-called bulletproof coffee and salad dressings, but essentially it is a 'healthy' fat which is contained in large quantities in coconut oil. They basically extract it by putting coconut oil in a centrifuge and it separates MCT Oil out. So why is it special?

MCT is an abbreviation for medium-length chain triglycerides. Due to their shorter length, MCTs are easily digested and have many health benefits which are linked to the way your body processes these fats.

MCT Oil has been shown to increase the release of two hormones that promote the feeling of fullness in the body: Peptide YY and leptin. One study found that people taking two tablespoons of MCT Oil as part of their breakfast ended up eating less food for lunch compared to those taking coconut oil. Now you're probably going to be skipping breakfast anyway, but you get the point.

Additionally, taking MCT Oil has been shown to significantly reduce body weight and waist circumference. Researchers even report that it could help prevent obesity.

MCT Oil has about 10% fewer calories than long-chain triglycerides (LCTs), which are found in foods such as olive oil, nuts and avocados; and your body also processes MCTs differently, which may help you burn calories more efficiently. Your body can use MCT Oil as an instant source of energy, making it unnecessary to store fat for this purpose. MCTs can be converted into ketones, which are produced from the breakdown of fat when carb intake is low. If you're following this way of eating, which is very low in carbs yet high in fat, then taking MCT Oil can help you stay in the fat-burning state of ketosis.

Also, your gut environment, i.e. flora and biome, is very important when it comes to your weight. MCT Oil can help optimise the growth of good bacteria and support the gut lining, which in turn could also help you lose weight.

Due to their shorter chain length, MCTs travel straight from the gut to the liver and do not require bile to break down(as is the case in longer-chain fats), so they can be an instant source of energy that can also be used to fuel your brain – which is not a bad thing as your brain will be running on fat and not sugar for energy!

In the liver, the fats are broken down to be either used as fuel or stored as body fat and since MCTs easily enter your cells without being broken down, they can be used as an immediate source of energy.

MCTs can also be converted into ketones in the liver – which pass through your blood-brain barrier, making them a convenient source of energy for your brain cells. Nice!

MCT Oil has become popular with athletes – as during exercise, lactic acid levels build up and cause muscle soreness in recovery, or DOMS (delayed onset muscle soreness) as we know it. So why is that relevant for us? Well now that we're going to be walking or running 30 minutes a day we don't want to feel sore as a result, so we can keep up our momentum. On top of that, one study found that taking the MCT Oil before exercise might help you use more fat instead of carbs for energy which might help if you are in transition or are comfortable with a very small amount of carbs in your diet anyway, such as I am.

There's evidence that as MCTs promote production of ketones they also have a beneficial effect for epilepsy in the same way that a ketogenic diet does. One test-tube study showed that the MCT capric acid improved seizure control better than a widespread anti-epileptic drug, so again MCTs and ketones are good for brain function. Indeed with Alzheimer's disease, one study found that a single dose of MCTs improved short-term cognition in 20 people with Alzheimer's disease with a certain associated gene type.

While genetic factors obviously play a role, evidence suggests that 20 to 70 grams of supplemental MCT Oil that includes caprylic or capric acid can modestly improve the symptoms of mild-to-moderate Alzheimer's.

Due to the caprylic and capric oils and lauric acid in MCTs, they have been shown to have antimicrobial and anti-fungal effects with coconut oil having been shown to reduce the growth of Candida albicans by 25%. This is a common yeast that can cause thrush and various skin infections.

If that's not enough, there is even some research on MCTs' effect on immune support; however that has been conducted via test-tube or animal studies. High quality human studies are needed before stronger conclusions can be made; but in the light of Covid-19 and the need for a strong immune system to combat the ever-mutating viruses out there, I'm willing to take the gamble.

When it comes to the effects on your weight, MCT Oil has been shown to support weight and fat loss. A study of 24 overweight men found that taking MCT Oil combined with phytosterols and flaxseed oil for 29 days reduced total cholesterol by 12.5%. However, when olive oil was used instead, the reduction was only 4.7%. The same study also found better reductions in LDL or 'bad' cholesterol when the MCT Oil mixture was added to their diet and it also increased the production of heart-protective HDL or 'good' cholesterol, whilst reducing inflammatory markers that increase the risk of heart disease. That is exactly the type of 're-composition' of cholesterol that we are looking for. MCT Oil could have many benefits and very few of the risks.

So to summarise, MCT promotes weight loss; reduces body fat; increases fullness; potentially improves your gut environment; is a great source of energy; may fight bacterial growth; help protects your heart; and aids in managing diabetes, Alzheimer's disease, epilepsy and autism. You can see why I have now introduced MCT into the plan of attack.

As long as you keep to one to two tablespoons per day and use it to supplement your diet, any negative side effects are negligible. Now putting oil in your coffee makes it a bit yuck in my opinion; however there are emulsified versions which mean you can add it to your coffee without feeling like you've drunk an oil slick (I recently bought a powdered version from my local health food store which I now use as my coffee creamer).

Now that we're talking about fats and how they are treated by the body, let's talk about:

Cholesterol

This word strikes fear into the hearts of mice and men! By the time you get to your 40s you know that cholesterol is the fat delivered into your bloodstream by your liver. There is bad cholesterol (LDL) and good cholesterol (HDL) and there are also triglycerides which are a type of fat (lipid) found in our blood. When you eat, your body converts any calories it doesn't need to use right away into triglycerides. The triglycerides are stored in your fat cells. Later, hormones release triglycerides for energy between meals. High triglycerides and levels of LDL are indicators of how likely you are to have clogged arteries and therefore be at risk of a heart attack.

However there is increasing evidence to show that your levels of LDL are much more influenced by your genetics than might have been imagined, and so a far more effective indicator would be the ratio between your HDL and your triglycerides. Essentially the closer that ratio is to 1:1 the better you are.

Which means that it's not the overall amount of cholesterol that is crucial but the type and the mode in which you use and store your fats. This is important, as studies have shown a correlation linking an 'overall' low cholesterol diet with degenerative brain conditions such as dementia and Alzheimer's, which also seems to correlate to its prevalence in recent times in exact proportions to the rise of the standard American diet and 'low-fat' craze.

So to conclude, don't be afraid of good natural fats and oils. Stay away from trans fats which exist in processed foods. Add in a little MCT if you feel inclined and over time your blood-work should improve as mine did. My own ratio came back to near 1:1 after some 10 years of it having been as high as 5:1 at its worst … yikes!

After nearly 18 months to two years of strict keto and then becoming a lazy beef-eater (carnivore), I had my first blood tests in early 2020! Can't say I wasn't nervous after eating more fatty steak and cheese that any man should. The results were triglycerides normal for the first time in 10 years. HDL (healthy cholesterols) up! LDL a bit up but not significantly. Overall cholesterols same. GGT fatty liver indicators (not shown) were also normal for the first time in 15 years. All coinciding with approximately 30kg of weight loss. So, draw your own conclusions. However, the doctor asked for MY advice on losing a few pounds. I couldn't believe it.

```
LIPIDS AND HDL

Date                 15/05/12  15/01/16  08/12/16  30/01/20
Time F-Fast          1200      1230 F    1400 F    1123 F
Lab ID               232699582 246250622 262310211 278603978 Units      Reference

Status               Random    Fasting   Fasting   Fasting
Cholesterol          5.0       H 6.2     H 6.5     H 6.5    mmol/L      (3.9-5.5)
Triglycerides        H 2.8     H 5.1     H 4.0     1.5      mmol/L      (0.5-1.7)
HDL Chol.                      0.9       1.1       1.3      mmol/L      (0.8-1.5)
LDL Chol.                                H 3.6     H 4.5    mmol/L      (1.7-3.5)

Comments on Collection 30/01/20 1123 F:
According to current guidelines (Position Statement 2005),
suggested targets are:
   HDL Cholesterol      >1.0 mmol/L
   LDL Cholesterol      <2.0 mmol/L (for patients at high risk)
                        <2.5 mmol/L (for patients at lower risk)
   Triglycerides        <1.5 mmol/L

Date                 15/05/12  08/12/16  30/01/20
                     1200      1400 F    1123 F
```

CHAPTER 5

EXERCISE –
MOVE YOUR BODY
AND FORGET THE GYM

We know that activity and exercise improves and regulates a whole host of things in our body. Mood, circulation, appetite etc. There are short-term benefits, and they are all obvious to see. However the longer-term benefits which impact on your longevity are perhaps not so obvious.

There is a massive correlation between an early death and lack of mobility. Any nursing home staff will tell you that as soon as a resident loses their mobility they go downhill much faster. Frailty is a major factor, but what is frailty? In a word ... weakness. Or to be more precise: loss of muscle-mass and physical strength, and lack of flexibility and range of movement. This is brought about by an escalating acceptance of a sedentary lifestyle, until eventually the sofa and a cup of tea is your prison rather than your comfort.

This frailty or weakness is directly measurable in terms of lean muscle mass. Without it you can't move about, let alone exercise. We all know people who are 'old beyond their years' and a lot of that is their physicality. So building some solid muscle is not a question of having bulging biceps but actually about building a foundation to allow you to live longer, and have a better quality of life. I'll call out the vegans here because each one I've met stereotypically looks somewhat weak and lacking in energy (and yes, I know there are exceptions).

So we all know that doing more exercise is a good thing but like our diet in modern times we've been fed a load of similarly confusing misinformation. Starting with marketing for gym memberships (only to be beaten, in their evil genius to strip you of your cash, by being sold bottled water), and finishing with a lot of confusion as you get older about supplements, heart rates and every other fitness gadget you can imagine.

Let's start with a few facts – Good ones!

The world seems to be obsessed with a flat stomach as a benchmark of weight loss achievement, and rightly so. Waist circumference is a reliable indicator of visceral fat (if you don't know what that is, read on) and overall health. For men and women that means abs. But in truth, we already have them! Yay! We can all go back to bed now. No seriously, we all have a functional six-pack hiding in there somewhere underneath several layers of belly fat. Your abs are already in perfectly good working order, as without them you simply wouldn't be able to stand up … you'd collapse like a jellyfish. Your core muscles stabilise almost all your movements and are some of the strongest muscle groups in your body. They could probably be stronger, and they most likely aren't very toned; but believe me, they are there. You just need to tease them out a little.

Just think about the weight they carry (especially if you're overweight) and the job they do. The idea that 'I don't have abs' or 'core muscles' is ridiculous. The real issue is you can't see them and they might be quite weak. In fact depending on your physiology and genetics you may never have seen them – and furthermore, you perhaps never will. You get a peek of them if your body fat is about 12% to 14% and you'll see some clear definition if they are toned and have about 5% body fat. Exercise in the context of this book is not about your superficial exterior but rather about what it looks like on the inside.

Instead of thinking about abs and a flat stomach, your focus should be on thinking about your 'external' fat as a reflection of your 'internal' fat!

So you have a belly or a spare tyre … big deal. Like I said most people are actually fairly comfortable with their appearance even though we'd all like to look better. However, there is a more important correlation when you look at that spare tyre, namely that it is a reflection of the amount of fat that is surrounding your vital organs, called visceral fat.

Fat around your heart, lungs, etc causes all manner of cardiovascular diseases and is the leading cause of death in the world (cough … Covid-19). Fatty liver causes sluggish metabolic function and stops your body from eliminating toxins. In fact, fat surrounding any organs – heart, liver, kidneys, spleen, lungs – is not going to help them function. Not a nice image. But this is the reality.

Any exercise we are talking about is aimed at the reduction of this fat, the fat you can't see. A six-pack, or flat tummy, might be what you're after; but that is a by-product of this ultimate goal.

Okay, but how much exercise, and what sort?

What sort of exercise should you be doing? Everyone's different and you now know that what works for one person doesn't work for someone else. You may have medical or metabolic issues, you may have injuries or physical limitations. That's all fine, but none of that is stopping you from taking a WALK (or a swim, or a cycle). The reason I emphasise walking (leading on to running) is that it needs no equipment compared to cycling, and it is always available; and even swimming needs access to facilities unless you are lucky enough to live by the water and have a good climate.

Walking, running, jumping and climbing are fundamentally what our bodies are designed to do – but like the childhood adage, 'don't run before you can walk', you have to start at the beginning and gradually adapt, and work your way up. From a health point of view walking delivers nearly all the benefits you need, but running gives you greater cardio resistance and respiratory health which is never more important than now to accelerate weight loss and health recovery. However walking is the gateway drug to more vigorous exercise.

In terms of building a micro-habit to include walking, it's easy. Just introduce a 30-minute brisk walk into your day, every day. Then in order to transition to running every other day, introducing running for two (just two) of those minutes, or more if you're able. Then increase by a further two minutes every day that you run, until you are running for 30 minutes every other day. This should take you no longer than one month to achieve – but if it takes longer, it takes longer.

At the point of comfortably running 30 minutes, you can extend to 40 minutes if you want, but no more than that. Why? Simply, we are NOT training to be athletes! Do not let competitiveness introduce the element of over-training and inevitable injury which will set you back. From personal experience, it easily happens; and as you feel better the temptation is to go a little harder, a little faster, a little further – but we are not in competition mode here.

Sure, challenge yourself; but we are in an 'achieve and maintain' mode. It looks like this:

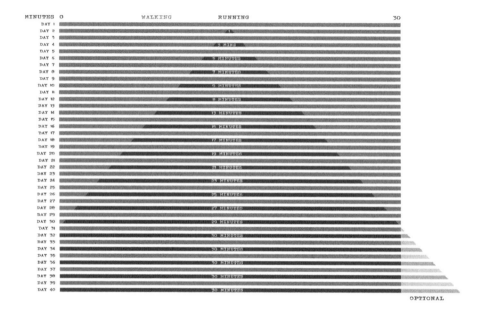

I would also recommend a running app such as Nike Run Club to keep track of your progress, but equally a Fitbit or any other technology that keeps track and engages you with building your daily habit.

If you are older or physically unable to run, then a brisk walk will do the trick, 100%. As mentioned, this delivers the vast majority of benefits and women on the whole are much better at taking a walk then men who often will opt for higher impact, more competitive options. The benefit of walking is that it's gentle. Low impact, and gentle on your heart. It's also gentle on your mind, and allows a bit of space. Walking meditation is a good thing and there are plenty of good downloads available to make a walk more than just moving your body.

If you're one of those people who think walking and running are boring, yeah, maybe you're right …. so, put some music on and do it anyway. If you have a dog, lucky you; the dog will thank you for it too. The truth is for our purposes we don't need to become marathon runners/endurance cyclists and spend hours on a treadmill, unless we grow to love it of course; but we do need a bit of cardio-vascular activity to activate all the hormones and body mechanisms which come with some light activity. Again, we are looking to stimulate the body's natural responses, become stronger, and build some lean body mass in the form of muscle – which will keep us functional and healthy.

What about the gym?

Gyms as we know them are a very recent invention. They simply didn't exist as we know them until the last 70 years or so, and yet our physical condition as a population has deteriorated almost in equal measure. No surprise!

Low-intensity, low-impact exercises such as walking, jogging, swimming and more recently cycling have been around forever, as has sport! Long walks, as a form of exercise and meditation/self-reflection, have been around since our existence. In the past, before cars, holidays were often in the guise of pilgrimages – which involved walking a path. In addition, it could be argued that a brisk walk is preferable to even jogging, as it would typically put you in a heart rate zone of 120 to 140 beats per minute, which is the 'fat-burning' zone and is lower impact.

Let's have a look at the modern gym as it has a few characteristics, good and bad, which are interesting – but not for obvious reasons. The main characteristics of why a gym CAN work are not to do with the exercise that takes place in it. Once you've joined a gym, the reason you go is because you've paid the money and you're not going to waste it! Hence why the gyms offer contracts and plans, although the tide is turning against them with increased competition. However the point is this: The membership is a 'call to account'.

The reason people find a personal trainer effective is not because we don't know how to do a push-up, but rather we have made a social appointment to meet someone, in this case our trainer (but it could equally be a friend), to exercise – and this has created a social obligation or contract to turn up! That's what you're really paying for – an appointment!

Now you could argue that if that were the case you make an appointment in your calendar to exercise and that would be that. However it is breaking the social contract and letting someone down if you don't turn up, that is the motivation to get you moving. For example you are far more likely to abandon a solo practice session of hitting tennis balls against a wall than to abandon a prearranged tennis match with your opponent. The concept is essentially an accountability partner.

To be fair, gyms have gotten a lot better and more of their focus is increasingly on group classes including things like yoga that introduce a social element which is a plus; but still, basic exercise is not something you have to pay for. It's free! Much like the water out of the tap!

Doing 15 minutes of stretching and going for a 30-minute walk does not require a direct debit. That is to say that exercise does not have a barrier to entry … and going to the gym is not essential, unless of course you enjoy it.

There is another drawback to the gym, especially for men. At the gym the group classes are predominantly the domain of the females who all attack synchronised routines; and although there are a few guys, it can make you feel like an uncoordinated fool, as you bounce your gut around next to some toned gym bunny who is way fitter than you and knows her left from her right. Although to be fair the recent trend for HIIT, spin and boxing based group classes is breaking down the gender divides.

For men who are NOT gym people (which is mainly who we are talking to here) there is a tendency to confine ourselves to the machines! But with no real sustained cardio routine, guys hit the treadmills and rowing machines for a bit before getting bored and playing with the free weights and weight machines, before getting bored! This is the ultimate half-arsed gym experience. We've all been there, and it's as boring as it is predictable.

So unless you have managed to make the gym into a positive experience (which it can be) by making it social, or going with a friend, or breaking through and becoming a group class junkie, or suddenly becoming so self-motivated that you work through your reps and sets like a champion (in which case why are you reading this book?), then this is all you really need to progress.

> **Walking, jogging, push-ups and sit-ups, and variations thereof. By introducing progressive levels and variations of those four things, you have EVERYTHING covered.**

At the end of this section are some diagrams which show variations of each, and I might get round to posting some YouTube videos to show some variations and 'next level' stuff to address specific areas which I think might be useful. It's nothing complicated. It doesn't have to be!

The genius of these exercises is that, on the whole, they are multi-activational exercises ... i.e. they work a lot of different muscle groups at once. A push-up for example works your core, your upper and lower back, shoulders, tricep, and so on. All the others do the same and when you add small variations you change the muscle groups to ensure no part of you gets left behind. Do not worry too much about legs, squats etc as regular walking and running will work your lower body, although a bit of skipping and jumping never hurt anybody. In fact IF you can adopt a skipping routine and you can stick with it, 'rope' is THE go-to cardio workout for boxers and it has the added benefit of being able to be done indoors virtually anywhere. Not a bad option in these times where we are dealing with the prospect of periods of quarantine perhaps becoming a fact of life.

In order to make a successful new exercise habit, it has to be easy and simple and you have to attach it to an old existing habit. The problem with exercise habits is we are too ambitious and too impatient. A five-minute walk leads to a 10-minute walk and so on. If running is your thing there are apps and podcasts like 'couch to 5k' with guided coaching telling you when to run and walk and so on. Embrace a bit of technology! One push-up leads to two etc. Can't even do one? Drop to your knees and do a half! Start small. Very small! A new routine when repeated for approximately three weeks cuts a new neural pathway and will become easy to ingrain as a new habit... so push through and persevere for those first three weeks. It'll soon get easier.

Don't forget if you're overweight, and especially if you're very overweight, the load that you are working with is significant. For example, take the simple push-up. Imagine some guy in perfect condition who weighs 75kg (12 stone) and does 10 push-ups. He is essentially pushing that weight up on his arms and shoulders. Now take you (or me, for that matter … I'm a fairly average stocky muscular six-foot frame who at the start of this book was over 120kg or almost 19 stone). So at that time I was pushing an extra six stone or 40kg for that one push-up. I guarantee you that if we took a suitcase weighing 40kg and put it on that imaginary guy, he may not even be able to do a single push-up either! So you have to adapt to your weight, relative load, and ability, and make this a manageable exercise that you can start to be consistent with.

The point is that we are aiming for a level of medium resistance. Not a linear or arbitrary number of push-ups, sit-ups etc. Look at the exercise that you are attempting, find a variation of it that gives you light to medium resistance, and aim to do 20! You really don't need to do any more than that to have a good effect on your body composition over time. There is research to suggest that the optimal number would be to do 12 to 15, when properly executed and so on; however 20 is a good round number so until you are ready to start working out your own routine: 20 of everything!

Consistency and Persistence!!

Similarly with walking and running (and I should say swimming if you can) instead of measuring distance rather measure your walks or runs in time. Forget five kilometres and instead walk/run 20 minutes out and 20 minutes back with light to medium intensity. A brisk walk, interspersed with a light jog. You get the picture.

Light to medium intensity is a great guidance for all your exercise. While there is always a new research fad which says that exercising at 1,000% for one minute a week will stop you getting dementia, the truth is that it's not going to help you squeeze into your tight jeans. HIIT or high intensity interval training may be the latest rage, and it works, absolutely; but it also has a much higher risk profile for injury for middle-agers. Also muscle soreness is a factor and therefore it's less likely to be something you will want to do regularly as a matter of habit, especially at the beginning when you are carrying a lot of weight. So leave that stuff for later, if you want, when you have built up a base level of fitness and have ditched your 'immediate' weight.

I was out having a jog once with a friend and saw a couple of very overweight guys doing sprint training! Why? I didn't know whether to stay in case an ambulance was needed or bet with my friend on who was going to pull a hammy first! And you don't need to lift heavy weights or do endless leg-burning squats and lunges. To get it straight… **Pain Is Not Progress** for our purposes, although there is nothing wrong with pushing yourself to get moving. Some resistance IS needed to build some strength, but this is and always will be provided by your own body weight.

You probably have heard of aerobic exercise but may not have heard of anaerobic exercise. In simple terms I like to think about it like this: Aerobic makes you run faster; anaerobic makes you run longer. Anaerobic burns fat, whereas aerobic builds strength. We need a bit of both, but a 'fat-burning zone' is a fairly low intensity rate of exercise delivered by something like a brisk walk or a light jog. Basically you want to get up a light sweat and maintain it for 30 minutes.

For the purposes of this book we are looking to decrease the bulk of our bodies, not start body building and become even more huge. That's not to be confused with building some healthy toned muscle mass, and functional strength. Overdoing it might actually be counterproductive and increase your risk of injury. So adapt to your age and stay within your level of ability. We are looking for an improvement in body composition.

If you have lost 10 to 15 kilograms (20 to 30 pounds or a few stone) and you want to increase the resistance and intensity of your exercise, then that gradual change will come naturally. So again, start small and don't rush it. The benefits will be by-products, as will your gradual adaptation to the new you, and you will have to increase your level of exercise to maintain your medium resistance and intensity of exercise. It is a positive adaptation syndrome.

So here's a simple little workout that will achieve everything needed to keep your muscle mass up, and change the composition and shape of your body. All of the following should be adapted to your ability and intensity.

20 push-ups
20 winged crunches
20 knee touches (micro sit-ups)
20 bench dips or reverse row pull-ups
1 minute plank
30 second side plank each side
20 squats (if you feel you are weak in the lower body)

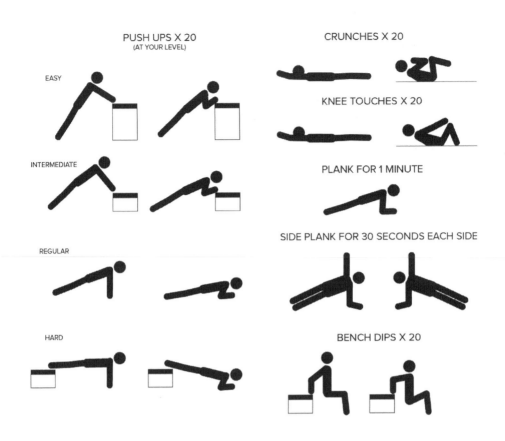

PUSH UPS X 20
(AT YOUR LEVEL)

EASY

INTERMEDIATE

REGULAR

HARD

CRUNCHES X 20

KNEE TOUCHES X 20

PLANK FOR 1 MINUTE

SIDE PLANK FOR 30 SECONDS EACH SIDE

BENCH DIPS X 20

That should take five to six minutes and it constitutes a set. THAT'S IT! Together with your walk or run and a little stretching after, you should be done in 45 minutes. If you're feeling fitter, recover for a minute and repeat the exercise component.

It goes without saying. Warm up for five minutes before exercise and stretch down for five minutes after. Flexibility and injury prevention is the goal. Incidentally, as you start to bring some muscle into your new habits you will come to a point where weight loss hits a plateau. More on that later, but as we put on some muscle (which weighs more than fat), you'll notice body composition changes more than those numbers on the bathroom scales. So don't get too neurotic about the bathroom scales.

CHAPTER 6

THE SECRET SAUCE –
'PUTTING IT ALL TOGETHER'

The trick to achieving and maintaining progress is simple: You must **COMBINE** the three strategies outlined so far: A low-carb eating plan/intermittent fasting/moderate exercise (including a 30-minute walk/run).

To lose weight fast and make a rapid transformation, do three out of three.

To maintain and make slow progress, do two out of three – but be strict about it.

For instance, if I can't exercise for whatever reason, I will be stricter and compensate with my fasting and way of eating; if it's not practical to avoid carbs for a period, I'll be more strict with my intermittent fasting and make sure I do some solid exercise every day; and so on. It looks like this:

	FASTING		KETO > CARNIVORE DIET		EXERCISE
MAINTANENCE	✓	OR	✓	AND	JUST WALKING
PROGRESS	✓	AND	✓	AND	JUST WALKING
OPTIMAL	✓	AND	✓	AND	FULL RUNNING + WORKOUT ROUTINE

In short, if you let one area slip, you can compensate with the others. However the best transformation comes by combining all three, and the results have a compounding effect. This really is the 'secret sauce' so to speak, and gives us the ability and flexibility to adapt through different life situations without complete abandonment of the whole plan.

My recommendation is to make fasting and way of eating your first priorities, as these will make the greatest difference – especially if exercise is difficult for whatever reason (not least because of the weight you might be carrying) – but in practice I interchange strategies and intensities depending on circumstances.

Commit to what you say you are going to do and have some integrity with yourself. Make your credo:

'Do what you say you are going to do, and do it when you said you were going to do it'.

Dealing with setbacks

In reality there will come a point in your journey when you've made some progress to begin with … however you'll hit a plateau, or you will encounter something that gets in your way. This could be an internal change such as boredom or compromise, or such as changing the goal posts; or an external change in circumstances, such as a new job, or new relationship, which puts some things in the 'too hard' basket and de-prioritises everything else.

This is possibly the most challenging element in the journey to losing weight and get healthy, especially after making some gains. The problem is this: We see some initial results and we're happy about them … great! However when the momentum starts to tail off we become discouraged and feel tempted to abandon the plan. This is the crucial stage because this is where we revert to what we perceive as 'normal'. This is what I call the 'yay, I'm thin, let's eat' mind-frame.

If you have successfully adapted though, your 'normal' will be largely the same low-carb plan you have been following for quite a while. In my case this was about the six-month mark. The key is to not throw the towel in, and to view 'maintenance' as a key stage in your journey. In doing this, we remove the expectation that we will have continual weight loss or some other improvement every week.

If the roadblock is something like boredom or repetition, if you've been eating the same chicken dinner for a few months, or been running the same run at the same time etc, it's inevitable, and for God's sake change it up a bit and introduce some variety within your eating and exercise plans. It's good for your nutrition, as well as your mind. Stay on it, as you don't want to establish an 'on-again, off-again' yo-yo routine.

Re-taking stock, and moving the goalposts

Measuring your progress and comparing yourself to where you were is important when you get to a point where you've made some progress. Moving the goalposts can be a two-sided coin. It can be a negative compromise, but at the same time if you move your goals further away as you achieve them this can be a way of self-motivating. In short, celebrate your micro-goals, but don't quit on your bigger picture.

Here is what you can expect: For me (and I would see these as typical of many) my micro-goals were to lose five kilograms at a time. My major milestone was to lose 25kg and get under 100kg and my ultimate goal is to get to 90kg because this is what I have defined as my ideal weight. I currently sit at 95kg and I continue to chip away at it, but I have basically achieved the health benefits I sought … so the journey continues. In short:

- I had sleep apnea and now I no longer even snore.
- I was extremely unfit, and now I comfortably run for 35 minutes or so every other day and feel fit from a respiratory health point of view.
- I felt weak and could barely do a few push-ups and now I do my little workout comfortably.
- My triglycerides were five times what they should have been and now they are normal for the first time in 20 years.
- My visceral fat score is now normal.
- I took painkillers and anti-inflammatories on a regular basis and now I take no medications!
- I had frequent injuries, pulled and strained muscles; and I am now injury free.
- I had significant plantar, knee, lower back and neck pain and now largely have no pain that warrants me taking a tablet or scheduling a therapeutic appointment of some sort.

This is not to be self-congratulatory, as I would describe myself as 'average'. Average in motivation, average in discipline, average in athleticism, and average in almost every other way.

This is to show that there is an easy path back from what are a very average set of conditions, which are making your life uncomfortable, and may be a precursor to more serious ill health and onset of disease.

This is the chance to address the situation before it gets worse and it's too late to do anything about it. So that's it!

What are you waiting for?

Frequently asked questions

I thought I'd cover a few other subjects which inevitably come up in relation to this approach from others, but including questions I had myself at the beginning of this journey.

Surely Vegetables contain a lot of MACRO nutrients that might be missed in a predominantly meat diet?

Meat is not just high in protein. It is also a source of many nutrients that are simply not available in plants. Meat provides B12, highly absorbable heme iron, pre-formed vitamins, all the essential amino acids, zinc, EPA, DHA, vitamin D, and vitamin K2, none of which are found in plant foods. It could be said that some antioxidants and things like Folate and vitamin C are the only things that are not provided by an exclusively meat-based diet. Everyone likes to say you'll get scurvy – but to be honest, a salad dressed with lemon juice and olive oil from time to time ain't going to kill you, and will easily cover that gap; but generally vitamin supplements are a good idea (making sure they do not contain saccharin or aspartame).

What about vitamins and supplements?

Essentially this guide is about possibly the easiest bio-hacking method possible. The advent of vitamin supplements might be a good correlation for increasing longevity and addressing basic vitamin deficiency caused illness since the post-war period. Practically speaking, a multi-vitamin might be a good catch-all; but in the context of this book, Bs, Cs and Ds are a far better idea as they are delivered in a much higher dose to cause some efficacy. A good B complex for mood, brain function, metabolism and endocrine system support generally. Approximately two to three grams per day of vitamin C for immune support seems optimal and two to three grams might appear to be a lot but it seems to be the best dose for bio-availability taken orally (according to Dr Rhonda Patrick) and is well documented for strengthening our immune system in its ability to combat viruses; and lastly vitamin D which is not just a vitamin, but also an important hormone which regulates all sorts of other genetic and cellular signals, and is essential for mood and immune support, and is suggested might be the missing link for combatting Covid-19, given the huge correlation of death amongst ethnic groups who are placed in vitamin D deficient environments.

Is beef and red meat better than other types of meats?

Even though other meats are quality sources of protein, beef simply blows a lot of other meats away in the nutrient department. It has significantly more B12, zinc, choline, iron and potassium. In terms of micro-nutrients, only chicken has more B3 than beef. Recommending people to reduce beef intake and replace it with vegetables is asking them to reduce the nutrient quality of their diets. However, it's a good idea to vary types of meat for variety and definitely include fish – especially smaller oily fish like sardines etc to get essential Omega 3s. A can of sardines is surely the ultimate portable power snack! sixy 4lis ♡

What about Fibre … Surely that much meat will give me constipation?

The reality is that stuffing huge quantities of fibre into our digestive tract actually makes it quite lazy, and more often than not causes wind, cramps and all sorts of problems. Hitler was famously a vegetarian and suffered from chronic constipation and laxative abuse. We stuff it in one end and we shift the same bulk through the other end. Bulking fibre like psyllium husk is not broken down, and just bulks up our stools. We're not inviting our colon to function as intended. Our digestive system contains strong bile acids, which entirely break down most non-vegetable matter. In fact it will break down meat to absorb almost everything and produce very little waste matter. In the course of eating an exclusively meat diet for over 12 months, I can tell you the amount of waste is very small; surprisingly so. What our colon does need to function however is plenty of water, electrolytes (aka salt), and sufficient fat content to stimulate proper bowel function. If constipation occurs, more fat in your diet is the answer nine times out of 10. More often than not, eggs and dairy can have a constipating effect – so cutting things like eggs out helps if it does happen. It has never been a problem in my experience, but everyone is different.

What about Fat?

Fat, especially saturated fat, has long been the convenient villain of the nutritional world. It has been blamed as the cause for all diseases and the reason we are obese, and that couldn't be more wrong.

Saturated fat is by far the most blamed as the main cause of high cholesterol and heart disease. It does raise cholesterol, and indeed typically raises overall cholesterol. The vilification of the type of fat that is primarily found in meat is completely unfounded.

The real culprit however is altered fats and chemicals found in processed foods, and what happens to fats when combined with a carbohydrate-rich environment. There is a lot of confusion between the two, deliberately banded together to vilify 'fats' as a whole, to the benefit of the sugar and wheat economy. The truth is that natural, good quality fats coming from animals are not harmful if taken in the right proportion to protein, and more importantly NOT combined with high sugar and carbohydrates. In fact, in my view, good quality animal fats are essential.

What about the environment?

You'll get this question a lot, when you start telling people what you're doing. The truth is our food system absent of animals simply does not work. Sustainable, regenerative agriculture involves animals playing a vital role. Synthetic fertilisers are destroying topsoil; and pesticides, which are completely normalised, are so poisonous that we really have to look at the effect they are having on the food chain. Animals may provide a solution to that problem.

Grazing enhances soil fertility, increases drought resistance, restores wildlife habitat, and sequesters carbon. Animals are a critical piece of creating a sustainable food system.

There is no doubt that intensive factory farming practices are barbaric and a real problem that we should all try to address, but let's not confuse the issues here. CO2 and methane production are only a problem in grain-fed cattle. Something they would never eat in the wild! Ruminant cattle (i.e. grass fed) and wild animals eaten by humans do not produce the gases that grain-fed, factory-farmed animals do. Just think about the inflammatory effect all that gluten does to humans and now feed a cow exclusively grain to get it as fat as possible to sell it at market. This is the real culprit behind gas emissions when people talk about intensive beef farming. Ruminant (more commonly called 'grass-fed' animals) actually create their own bio-diversity as they create a food chain of smaller animals as a by-product of their grazing habits.

Now, what about the environmental impact of vegetables? Unless you are growing them in your back garden, these same intensive farming factors apply to your vegetables too. The environmental impact of factory or intensive farmed vegetables is horrendous. From water usage to grow avocados to the destruction of Indonesian forests to grow palm oil, the list goes on. Not to mention that much non-seasonal fresh produce is flown in from all over the world and you have a carbon footprint unlike any other. So in short, buy local (i.e. nobody needs to buy lamb, or avocados, from across the planet when there is lamb in the next paddock), buy small, and buy fresh, and support your local livestock farmers. Whatever food you eat, don't over-consume and eat the best quality produce you can afford.

What does your current food plan look like?

Currently the day starts with a coffee (two Stevia sweeteners and a spoon of MCT Oil powder or heavy cream); soon after, a mug of beef bone broth with a teaspoon of butter in it. I'll repeat that throughout the day and add a few glasses of water until dinner time. For dinner some steak, half a dozen sausages or an equivalent amount of other meat. If I have a stew or curry I'll usually allow some onion or garlic for texture and finish with cream and ground almond-meal for thickening instead of flour. If I feel the need, I'll have an occasional small green salad made up of lettuce. If I want to bulk up my dinner I'll add a few eggs and if I'm still hungry, I'll have some cheese after dinner. I usually finish the day with a decaf coffee, and if I'm gonna drink then it's a bourbon on ice or in my coffee! That said, I have now quit alcohol altogether as it contributes a lot of excess calories that frankly I don't miss that much. I tend to eat at about 8.30pm'ish and finish about 9.30pm to 10.00pm – although I'm trying to eat earlier. Once a week or fortnight I will fast for 48 hours. Typically, I don't eat on Wednesdays. On those days, I just get by with coffee and broth. I can honestly say as long as I keep the broth going, I don't get hungry. I also use that day to have a rest day from any exercise if I feel I need to.

What does your daily exercise routine look like?

I walk and jog on alternate days, every day for about 35 to 45 minutes, maintaining a low to medium intensity. I avoid hills (although hills are better for fat burning), as I tend to get tight calves and I want to avoid injury. Every day, I do about 20 push-ups, 20 bench dips, 40 to 60 sit-ups including variations, and one minute regular and side plank which takes about five to 10 minutes. I've been doing more core work, because belly fat is stubborn and the last to leave the house.

Further reading and references

As mentioned this is not meant to be an overly-complicated peer reviewed scientific paper, nor is it meant to be aimed at those with extreme sensitivities and conditions (although in my view it'll most certainly help), or those who are fighting fit and don't need the help. Equally this is not to demonise any other diet or nutritional approach if it's working for you. Below are some options for you if you want to explore further.

Dr Jason Fung – https://thefastingmethod.com

He's a world-leading expert on therapeutic fasting and low carb for those with Type 2 diabetes.

Dr Shawn Baker MD – https://shawn-baker.com

Leading researcher, author of The Carnivore Code and exponent of the carnivore lifestyle. He is a giant ex-pro rugby player, crazy rower, orthopaedic surgeon and example of maintaining great results at the plus-50 age bracket and for athletic performance. No-one can say he is your typical average Joe. He is not! MeatRX is his paid platform, but a lot of his info is freely available.

Dr Kaayla Daniel, Ph.D — https://youtu.be/3ZrgETZzb0A

Dr Daniel (aka The Broth Lady) is co-author of 'Nourishing Broth: An Old-Fashioned Remedy for a Modern World' with her PhD in Nutritional Sciences and Anti-Ageing Therapies. Her TED Talk on Bone Broth and Health is everything you want to know and more.

Mikhaila Peterson — https://mikhailapeterson.com

Those who are suffering acute sensitivities should read and follow this very inspiring young woman who has overcome severe health problems (both physical and psychological) through an extreme version of this way of eating called the Lion Diet.

Dr Jordan B Peterson — https://www.jordanbpeterson.com

Famous psychologist, author of '12 Rules for Life' and university professor. If you want to address the body, first you must address the mind. An amazing guy who distils psycho-babble into practical wisdom for the rest of us. He has been through his own trials and tribulations so he's not one to preach from an ivory tower. Oh yeah … he's also the father of the aforementioned Mikhaila Peterson.

Jeff Cavaliere — https://athleanx.com

Jeff is a trainer and fitness guru. Much of his work is focused on body weight and callisthenics. If you want to take your training to the next level, his paid program is Athlean X – but like all of the above he puts a lot of free content up on YouTube.

That's it for now. I will address any further questions on the website in due course, and start some other content such as recipes and workout tips, and success stories etc. So … good luck. Keep with it and pretty soon you won't recognise yourself.

**Let me know how you get on at
www.thelazybeefeater.com**

Success Stories

These are just some of the amazing and consistent cases of people including myself following this way of eating combined with fasting and exercise.

Dean M (Yep, that's me!), 50 yrs old – London, UK

Starting weight: 125kg / 275lb / 19.5st
Current weight: 95kg / 210 lb / 15st
Ideal / target weight for my build is 90kg / 200lb / 14st

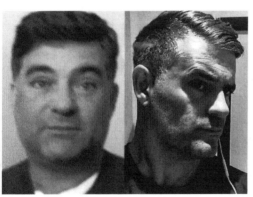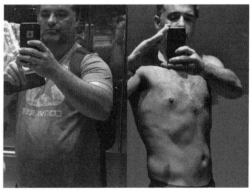

I started out on this way of eating approximately two years ago, starting with a lazy keto style of eating, then becoming progressively more strict, and in the last year becoming what I'd describe as lazy carnivore with approximately 90% to 95% of my food intake coming from unprocessed animal product, and introducing intermittent fasting thereby eating one meal a day. Once a week I do a 36 to 48 hour fast, eating dinner Tuesday night and then breaking my fast with breakfast on Thursday morning, with plenty of broth in between.

I do 35 to 45 minutes a day walking/running plus 10 to 15 minutes a day of body weight (callisthenics) as described. All are improvised to my own level of strength and ability, which varies.

My trigger to begin was poor sleep; snoring; pre-sleep apnea; aching knees, neck, lower back; and generally feeling puffy, bloated and dreadful – all the classic signs of inflammation. All my clothes were tight. Also I had some worrying blood test results indicating fatty liver and high triglycerides. My doctor was advising I see a cardiologist and predicting a prescription Statin. All of these things have been normalised.

My body composition has steadily and progressively improved and has been steadily maintained for over two years. I take no medication, and honestly feel better than I did in my 20s!

Josh A, 36 yrs old – Texas, USA

Starting weight: 168kg / 371lb / 26.5st (BMI of 51)
Current weight: 93kg / 205lb / 14.5st (BMI of 27)
Ideal weight approximately 86kg / 190lb / 13.6st with a BMI of <25

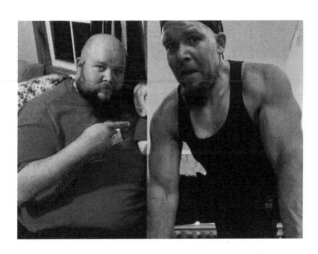

I've been on this current way of eating since a little over 16 months ago, starting with meat-based keto. After 15 months with good overall success I went full carnivore and started intermittent fasting (IF) routines and have been full carnivore/IF ever since.

For exercise I do some basic resistance training with weights, dumbbells, a curl bar and some plates etc, but about half of my workout routine is callisthenics, sit-ups, crunches, push-ups, pull-ups, etc. I walk 10-plus miles once a week. Every other night of the week is some form of training.

My particular trigger to begin my weight-loss journey was a Dept of Transport physical in mid-2017 where I was told I would lose my Commercial Licence if I did not change my weight/BMI. That was my tipping point. Over the course of that summer I researched the science behind weight loss and started keto in October 2017.

My health issues at the time were pre-hypertension, pre-diabetes Type 2 and borderline sleep apnea. My resting blood pressure averaged 145/95; it is now averaging 120/70. My haemoglobin A1c was 6.1; it is now 4.9. And I sleep like a baby!

I've maintained my weight loss for 2.5 years and counting. Still cutting body fat actually, though not losing weight because I am putting on lean mass to replace the body fat. My most recent goal set is a body fat percentage of under 14%. I am currently at 16% to 17%.

I easily feel like I was in my early 20s. It is AWESOME! And I will never stop. It simply works for my body.

Moira A, Brisbane, Australia

Down 30kg / 65lb / 4.5st

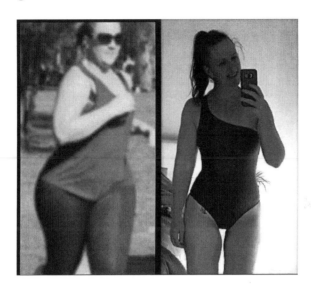

I decided to try this way of eating after my weight kept on going up and I was struggling to live with all-consuming anxiety. I had been working out at the gym three times a week; and as best I could, eating a 'balanced diet,' but it felt like my body wasn't responding to anything any more. I decided to give this way of eating a go because … what did I have to lose, really? From the first day my anxious worrying was replaced with calm and peacefulness. It was VERY obvious to me that the anxiety I was plagued with was gone. Whether it was some random placebo effect or just beginner's luck, it was enough to make me continue and stay on track.

The anxiety has not returned since, and a delightful side effect is that I have lost over 30kg since starting. I went from a size 16 to a size 6 (Australia) and completely changed my relationship with food.
Food used to always be about what I felt like. Going carnivore completely shifts that mindset and now I don't eat for feelings; I just eat to fuel myself when I feel hungry. It's so super simple.

As I continue on this path the benefits just keep stacking up; no adult acne, clear eyesight, boundless energy, reduced cellulite, stabilised moods, anxiety and depression diminished/gone; and I transformed into a perfect weight for my body.

I have kept this way of eating as simple as I could – because I know myself, and I am not the best at sticking to things if they are complex. I eat lean cuts of meat when hungry, I eat butter/cheese for fat and also consume bacon and eggs. I am now 90% carnivore. At the end of the day I have changed my relationship with food and can now trust my body to tell me what it needs. Generally I fast from the day before until lunch the next day, but I keep it flexible.

The simple handbook combining a few simple and adaptable strategies for enduring health and weight-loss. Specifically aimed at those who are in or approaching middle-age and are tired of fad diets, gyms, personal trainers, and going hungry. Rethink, what, how, and when you eat. Challenge the plant-based paradigm, and set yourself free.

www.thelazybeefeater.com

Printed in Great Britain
by Amazon